W9-AFC-052

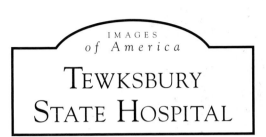

IMAGES
of America

TEWKSBURY
STATE HOSPITAL

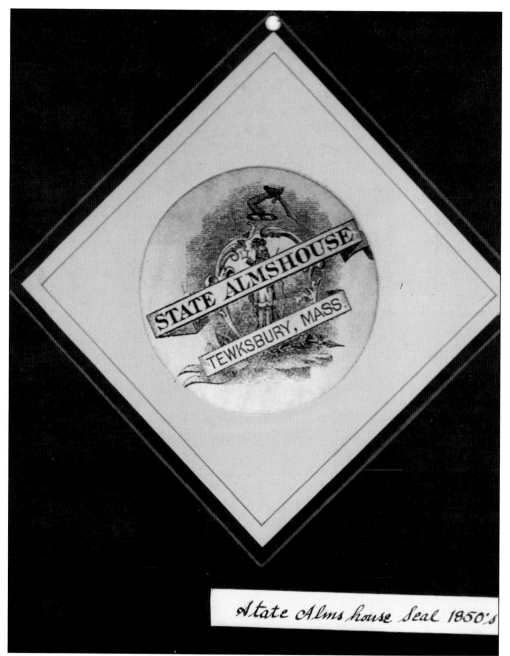

State Alms house Seal 1850's

At its founding, the seal of the State Almshouse at Tewksbury depicted the coat of arms of Massachusetts with the institutional name displayed across it. The almshouse seal would be seen for decades at the Tewksbury State Hospital, appearing on trinkets, furniture, and buildings throughout the campus. (Courtesy of the Public Health Museum.)

ON THE COVER: Pictured is the Female Hospital of the State Almshouse at Tewksbury in 1892, acknowledged at the time as the newest and most modern hospital in the United States. (Courtesy of the Public Health Museum.)

IMAGES
of America

TEWKSBURY
STATE HOSPITAL

Ashlynn Rickord Werner
and Jon Maynard

ARCADIA
PUBLISHING

Published by Arcadia Publishing
Charleston, South Carolina

Printed in the United States of America

Library of Congress Control Number: 2020951413

For all general information, please contact Arcadia Publishing:
Telephone 843-853-2070
Fax 843-853-0044
E-mail sales@arcadiapublishing.com
For customer service and orders:
Toll-Free 1-888-313-2665

Visit us on the Internet at www.arcadiapublishing.com

*To all who have contributed to the rich tapestry
of Tewksbury State Hospital.*

CONTENTS

ACKNOWLEDGMENTS

As the chief purveyors of the Tewksbury State Hospital collection, this book would not be possible without the Public Health Museum. Although the Tewksbury Hospital is still active, the Public Health Museum has become the repository for all items pertaining to the institution, from its early days as an almshouse to its present functions as a bustling campus for medical care and history. We wish to acknowledge members of the board of directors and museum volunteers, past and present, who shared their stories and insights about the Tewksbury State Hospital and actively preserved the photographs, objects, and records of the institution for the public to explore for decades to come.

All of the images in this volume appear courtesy of the Public Health Museum, except where noted.

We also would like to extend our thanks to the libraries, museums, archives, and individuals who permitted us to include their images in this publication in hopes of providing a most complete history of the Tewksbury State Hospital. We would also be remiss without extending a thank-you to the Tewksbury Historical Society for its support of this project, Michelle Halliwell for her proofreading and editing expertise, and our Arcadia Publishing team, Jeff Ruetsche and Caroline Anderson, for their guidance.

On a personal note, Ashlynn would like to thank her family for their support, especially her husband, Brad, and their dog Hampton for patience and encouragement throughout this whole process.

Introduction

The philosophy of this hospital is based primarily on the principle that regardless of race, creed or color, the care of each patient is given on an individual basis with respect to his every need. The general aim of our institution is to function in a most alive and alert manner, looking back when we can learn from the past, but constantly looking ahead, striving to preserve our vital and honored traditions but always moving with the mainstream to keep abreast of the acknowledged pace setters in health care.

—The Philosophy of Tewksbury Hospital, 1968

By 1852, when three state almshouses were commissioned, the commonwealth of Massachusetts had undergone a great change from an agrarian way of life to an industrialized society. Industrialization coincided with the need for a plentiful labor force, which in turn led to increased immigration. Although most found jobs in mills or factories, low wages and substandard living conditions caused much strife for those seeking a better opportunity in America. Many would wind up amid the public welfare system, and those without legal residence, mainly recent immigrants, could seek shelter in a state almshouse.

The State Almshouse at Tewksbury opened its doors on May 1, 1854, to serve paupers in northeastern Massachusetts. Constructed to house 500 persons, by the end of May, admissions climbed past 800, including maternity cases, infants and children, the insane, the acutely and chronically ill, alcoholics, persons with infectious diseases, and the indigent poor.

The year 1866 brought a classification change among state almshouse residents, with Tewksbury serving as "a receptacle of those who, through misfortune and poverty which they could not avoid, are compelled to receive, at the hands of the State, the living which their own hands could not earn," according to the Annual Report of 1886. Children were moved to Monson, and the able-bodied were sent to the State Workhouse at Bridgewater, leaving the sick and harmless insane to the custody of Tewksbury administrators. As the patient population changed, so too did the function of the institution.

The next two decades saw an expansion of the campus, both in terms of size and operations. Land was cultivated for farming and to raise livestock, new services were offered for the sick, and industrial therapy was affirmed as a therapeutic method of rehabilitation. When the almshouse came under the charge of a board of trustees in 1879, the expansion of medical services was further prioritized, solidifying the institution's future as a hospital.

Although the institution came under fire in 1883 for claims of neglect and deplorable conditions, much of the rumors were dismissed as the ravings of a governor seeking a presidential nomination, using the case against the State Almshouse at Tewksbury as a political ploy to seek mass approval. Unbeknownst to Gov. Benjamin Butler, the spectacle would actually benefit the institution, as the almshouse received renewed interest from the state in providing ample resources to ensure that the "accumulation of human misery, infirmity, disease and vice" would be kept to a minimum, according to the Annual Report of 1884.

The successive superintendents championed major building projects from the late 1800s through the early 1900s, coupled with great advancements in hospital management and in the care of the state's mentally and physically ill. During this time, the hospital's operations were departmentalized, and increasingly skilled staff were employed between men's and women's services, with many coming from the Training School for Nurses started in the 1880s. The expanded personnel were essential in operating the new asylum and hospital buildings, especially considering the growing prevalence of infectious diseases treated at the Tewksbury State Hospital.

With Robert Koch's discovery of the tubercle bacillus, the bacteria that caused tuberculosis, a greater effort was made by public health professionals to not only teach prevention methods, but also to provide "treatment" to tubercular patients. In the early 1900s, two hospitals were constructed on the outer edges of Tewksbury State Hospital to provide a place for ample rest and sunlight in a secluded environment away from the rest of the campus. Other patients with infectious diseases were also cared for in isolation wards, while the laboratory honed its skills in diagnosis and clinical treatment.

Whether under the guise of the almshouse ward, the insane department, or the hospital, patients were afforded opportunities for recreation and socialization. From religious services in the Old Chapel to spectating at the state infirmary baseball games, great care was taken to provide patients with a sense of community within an abnormal environment. For many, the entertainment acted as a ray of hope amid chronic ailments that could often restrict patients to a life of institutionalization.

By the mid-20th century, the Tewksbury State Hospital and Infirmary had peaked at almost 900 acres, over 50 buildings, and a daily staff of over 600. Yet, change would come in 1959 as a state departmental shift led to a reconfiguration of services and a new name. Subsequently known as the Tewksbury Hospital, the institution essentially became a chronic disease hospital, with those suffering from mental illness or infectious disease being transferred elsewhere. The specializations offered were broad with restorative services, an inhalation therapy department, obstetrics, and enhancements to long-standing services like the surgical department, the laboratory, and nursing care.

Today, the Tewksbury Hospital continues to offer a wide range of services for a diverse patient population within the Thomas J. Saunders Building. The broader campus structures are home to five state agencies, almost a dozen clinical programs, a therapeutic equestrian center, and a museum dedicated to the history of public health. The public library, schools, low-income housing, a community garden, and recreational facilities all occupy former state hospital land, interweaving the hospital history with the town of Tewksbury.

While the doors to most state institutions were shuttered in the latter half of the 20th century, Tewksbury State Hospital persevered. And over 165 years later, the institution continues to care for a myriad of Massachusetts citizens, paralleling the first residents admitted to the State Almshouse on May 1, 1854.

One

CARING FOR THE POOR

Poverty has seemed an inescapable blight to most governments since the beginning of civilization. As the ancient Greeks and Romans discussed the systematic treatment of the poor, so too did the early settlers of the United States. Throughout the colonial, provincial, and constitutional periods of the United States, members of individual towns were responsible for overseeing the condition and care of their poor. Disagreement was had, however, over the means of care provided to the impoverished. Founding father Benjamin Franklin spoke fervently on this issue. In his article "On the Price of Corn and Management of the Poor," Franklin wrote:

> I am for doing good to the poor, but I differ in opinion of the means. I think the best way of doing good to the poor, is not making them easy in poverty, but leading or driving them out of it. . . . There is no country in the world where so many provisions are established for them; so many hospitals to receive them when they are sick or lame, founded and maintained by voluntary charities; so many alms-houses for the aged of both sexes, together with a solemn general law made by the rich to subject their estates to a heavy tax for the support of the poor.

While Franklin was often a proponent of less government intervention into the welfare of the poor, many local officials felt escalating pressure as the impoverished became more prevalent, demanding further state involvement. Although the erection and maintenance of municipal workhouses and poorhouses can be traced to statutes enacted in the late 17th century, it was not until the statute of 1852, chapter 275, that Massachusetts took full responsibility for its "state paupers."

One distinct difference separated "state paupers" from paupers—the determination of settlement. Paupers had a legal residence in a town, city, or district, whereas state paupers did not. These "vagrants" were the financial responsibility of the commonwealth, and their care would be provided for at one of the three state institutions that opened in 1854.

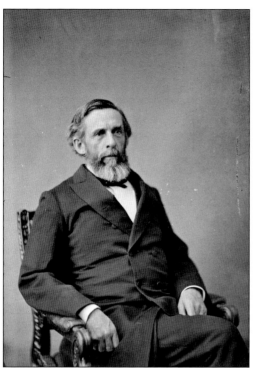

Upon the recommendation of the Joint Special Committee on Alien Passengers and State Paupers in 1852, the Massachusetts legislature authorized Gov. George S. Boutwell to appoint three commissioners to select three sites for the purpose of erecting almshouses that could accommodate 500 state paupers each. The commissioners believed that the expenses incurred to construct these institutions would be recouped within two years from immigration tax income, and the almshouses would become self-sufficient, thus financially beneficial to the state. (Courtesy of the Brady-Handy photograph collection, Prints and Photographs Division of the Library of Congress.)

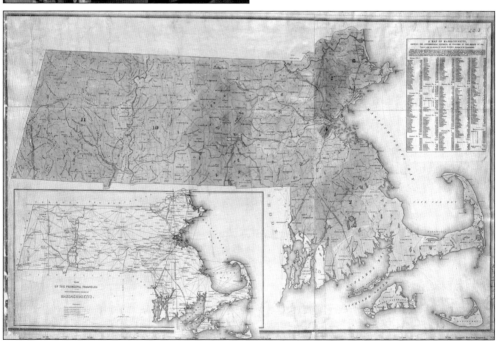

In selecting three sites, the commissioners were tasked with choosing a location within the counties of Bristol or Plymouth for one, the counties of Essex or Middlesex for another, and to the portion of the commonwealth west of the town of Brookfield for the third. The selected sites were to be in Bridgewater, Monson, and Tewksbury. (Courtesy of the Norman B. Leventhal Map & Education Center at the Boston Public Library.)

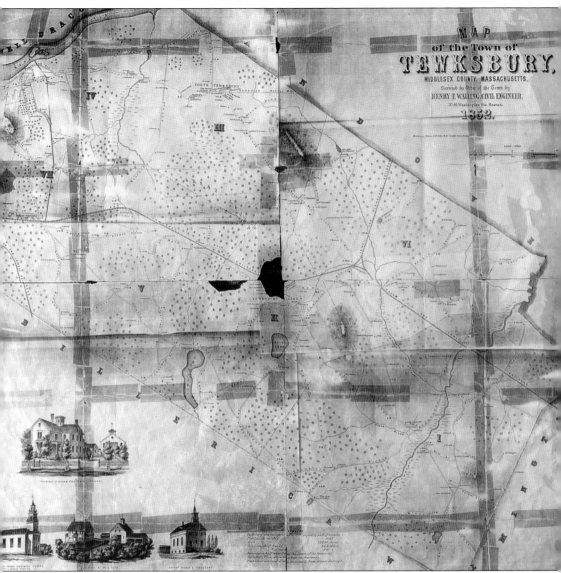

While evaluating potential locations for the new almshouses, the commissioners gave priority to sites that were in close proximity to railroad lines, had access to a healthy water source, possessed farmable land, and could be bought for a bargain. Tewksbury met each of these considerations. It was along the Lowell & Lawrence Railroad line, which converged with the Salem & Lowell Railroad about four miles east of the potential almshouse site. The Strongwater Brook passed through the proposed property, and the city of Tewksbury itself sat between the Concord and Merrimack Rivers, creating a natural richness for farming, albeit requiring pauper labor to best cultivate the reclaimed land in the early years. And lastly, the land was able to be purchased for a very low price. In total, roughly 142 acres were purchased in the town of Tewksbury for $3,423.59, about $24 per acre. (Courtesy of the Tewksbury Public Library.)

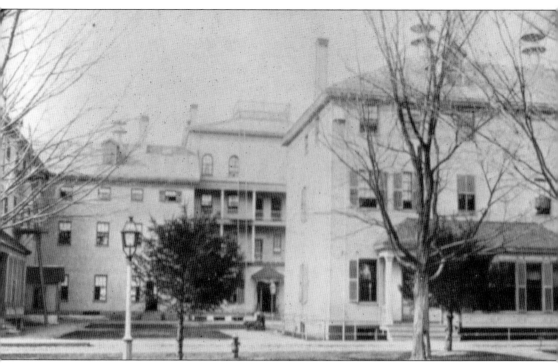

Financial accommodations were also required for the construction of the almshouse in Tewksbury. The commissioners accepted public bids for the erection of the building in the fall of 1852. Upon review of the bids, the price of construction was significantly higher than initially expected, with the contract being awarded to Albert Currier of Newburyport in the amount of $34,287, which was $15,000 over the initial projection. Cheaper building material was selected to keep the overall price down, while additional funds were needed to outfit the facility with furnishings for patients and staff. The legislature also appropriated funds to construct sheds, outhouses, an icehouse, and a tomb for the almshouse, although upon opening day, the institution was still unfinished.

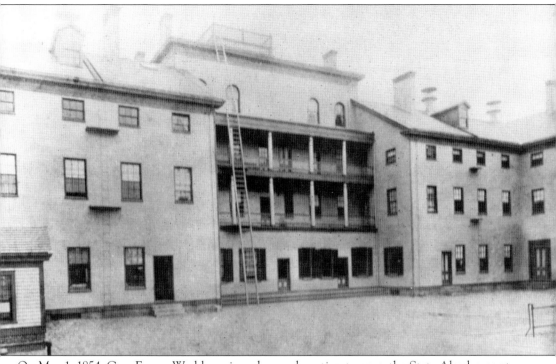

On May 1, 1854, Gov. Emory Washburn issued a proclamation to open the State Almshouse at Tewksbury. The original building in which the almshouse opened was constructed of wood. The commissioners tasked with erecting the three almshouses chose wood for the building's construction as it saved $26,462 in comparison to utilizing brick. The commissioners were conscious of the hazards with wood construction, but they believed the structure would suffice for 50 to 75 years. They decided to incur the additional expense of installing a slate roof and iron gutters instead of sawed shingles and wooden gutters, which would boost safety. The almshouse building was a U-shaped structure with four stories at the center and three stories on both wings. The center housed the administrative functions, and the wings housed males on one side and females on the other. Between the wings was a lush courtyard designed to be both majestic to the public and therapeutic for patients.

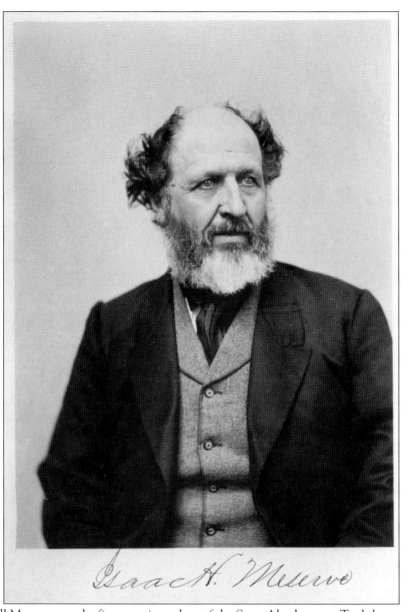

Isaac H. Meserve

Isaac Hall Meserve was the first superintendent of the State Almshouse at Tewksbury, although he was not new to this type of role. From 1842 to 1854, Meserve served as the superintendent of the Roxbury Almshouse before coming to Tewksbury. Under his leadership, most patients were employed about the almshouse either for housework, in the various shops, or tending to the farm. As superintendent, Meserve routinely called attention to the oversight of the children in the commonwealth's care. The 1855 Act Providing for the Classification of State Paupers passed by the general court mandated that state pauper children between the ages of five and sixteen be sent to the almshouse at Monson, but Meserve believed this to be problematic as parents incurred much trouble and expense to retrieve them from Monson. Thanks to Meserve and his almshouse colleagues strongly opposing this mandate, the general court repealed the act in May 1856 and allowed for children to be cared for at the almshouse in their respective district. (Courtesy of the State Library of Massachusetts.)

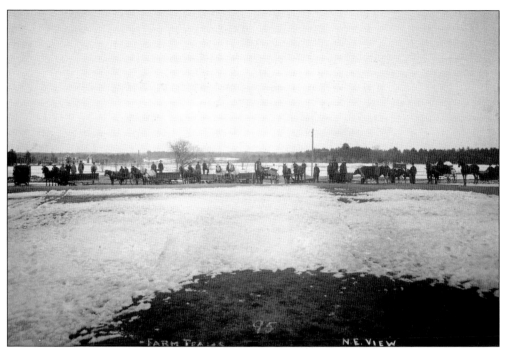

Within his first three years at Tewksbury, Meserve vastly improved the grounds and farmland. The farm, likened to the Sahara Desert in the early years, was brimming with trees, bushes, stumps, stones, and ploughed, sandy earth. Substantial blasting and removal of stone was completed, and the materials were reused to build roads and a stone fence around the yard. The cleared land was cultivated for the harvesting of grains and vegetables for the almshouse. (Courtesy of Harvard Art Museums/Fogg Museum, Transfer from the Carpenter Center for the Visual Arts, Social Museum Collection.)

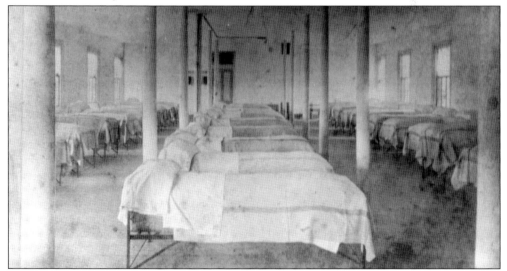

Unfortunately, the State Almshouse at Tewksbury faced overcrowding from the day it opened its doors in 1854. Originally built to house 500 paupers, on May 1 there were well over 500 persons waiting for admission. By the end of the first week, there were almost 700 paupers in state care, and by December 1, 1854, there had been 2,193 persons admitted to Tewksbury.

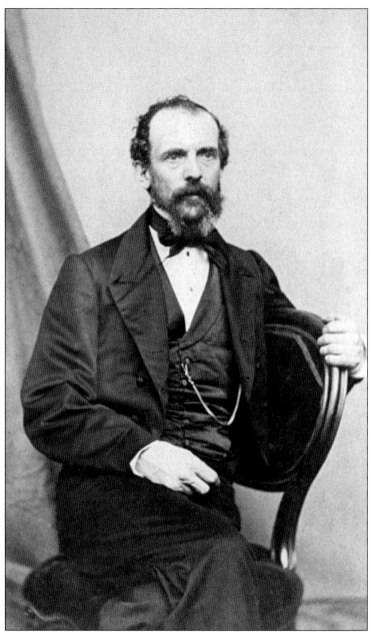

Disease was also quick to find the almshouse. Dr. Jonathan Brown, the first physician at Tewksbury, reported in the Annual Report of 1854 that two serious and fatal diseases had visited, cholera in May and June and "in October there appeared among the children an endemic gangrenous sore mouth, of singular virulence and fatality." A total of 161 paupers died between May 1 and December 1, 1854. By November 30, 1855, Dr. Brown noted that in the course of the year, 1,311 cases of sickness were reported in the hospital records, which excluded those that were treated in the regular wards when the hospital wards had exceeded capacity. Superintendent Meserve authorized the large room originally dedicated as the chapel to be converted for additional hospital accommodations. This need for more hospital space foreshadowed the almshouse's future as a leading medical facility for Massachusetts. (Courtesy of Buried By Time Photography Asylum Collection.)

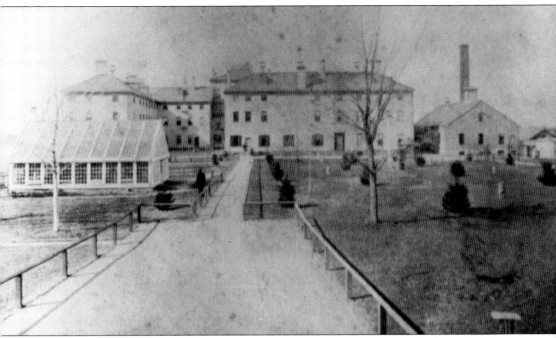

In May 1855, an appropriation of $12,000 was made to construct a kitchen independent from the main building. Previously, the kitchen was in the basement of the almshouse, and the administration was concerned about the possibility of a fire ravaging the wooden structure. The appropriated funds were used to build the cookery, which was connected by a covered passage to the main building. It was constructed of brick to quash fears of a fire breaking out. The building was 65 feet long and 43 feet wide, with the kitchen, a bakery, and food storage on the main floor. The attic was used for additional storage, and the basement became the laundry and drying room before a separate laundry building was constructed years later. The inmates of the almshouse were instrumental in the construction, having dug the cellar, transported building materials to the site, and laid the walls for the kitchen.

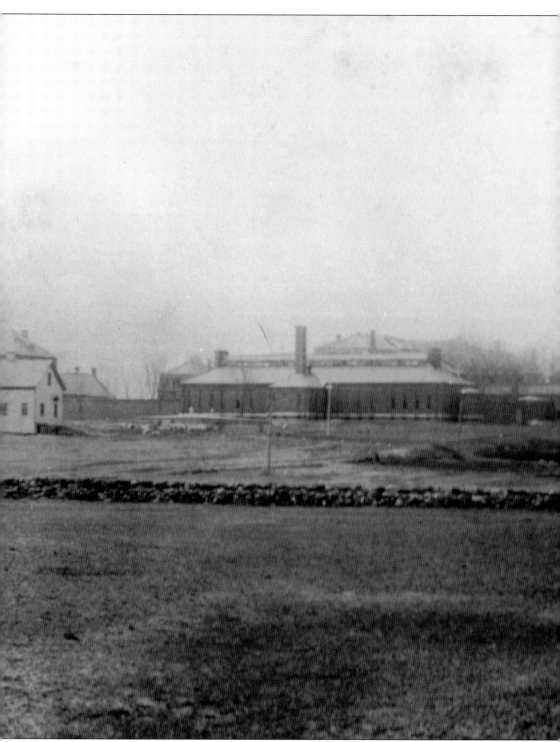

As admissions continued to rise, the need for further expansion became dire. Thomas J. Marsh, who became superintendent in 1858, led the charge of increasing the institutional capacity and providing more specialized care for the inmate population. Between 1860 and 1880, many

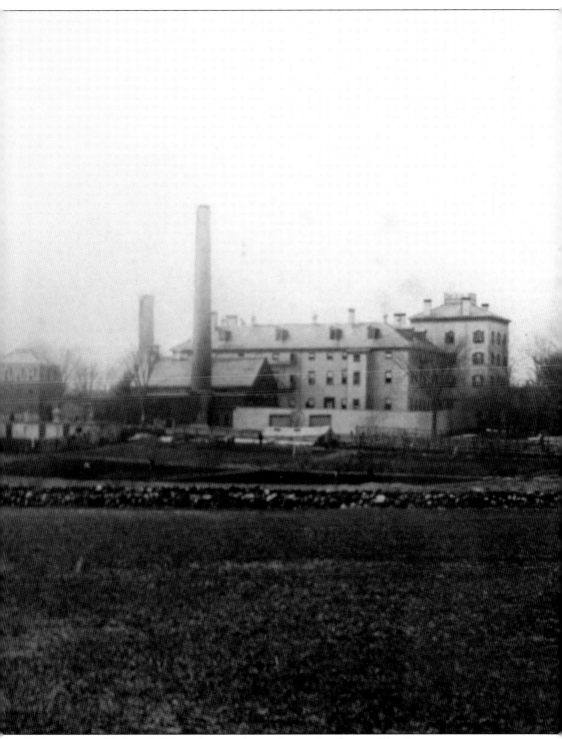

facilities were added, including infectious disease hospitals, a hospital for the insane, a reservoir, barn, and other outbuildings.

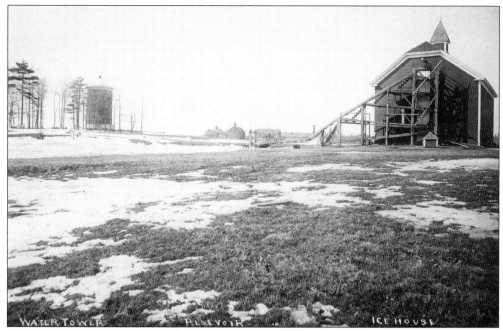

Convenient access to water was of constant concern to early almshouse administrators. An ample water supply was essential to power steam heat through the buildings and to protect the almshouse from fire. In 1868, the construction of a large reservoir was begun on the high land south of the campus to add to smaller reservoirs that were built previously. An icehouse would be added here in 1888. (Courtesy of Harvard Art Museums/Fogg Museum, Transfer from the Carpenter Center for the Visual Arts, Social Museum Collection.)

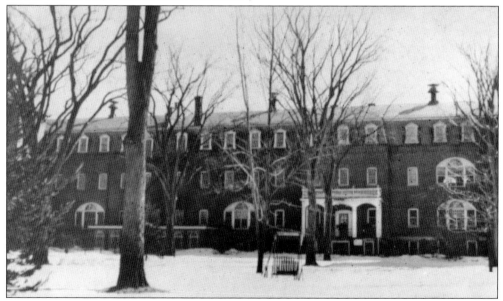

By 1860, sick inmates and the "harmless insane" made up the bulk of almshouse residents, and as early as 1861, calls for better accommodations for the mentally ill were made to Gov. John Andrew. This request was repeated for several years until sufficient funds were allocated in 1865 for the completion of the asylum to house the male and female harmless insane population.

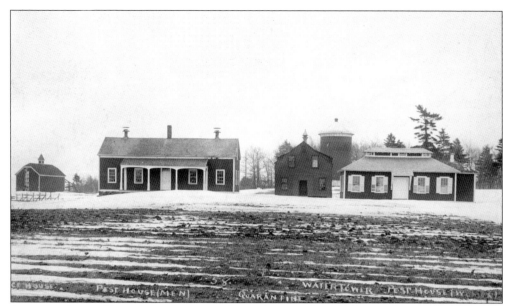

A new pesthouse, likened to a quarantine hospital, was built in 1861 to replace a farmhouse that was acquired with the purchase of the almshouse property in 1852. Superintendent Marsh noted that the farmhouse's appearance "excited the fears of the citizens, by reason of its peculiar location, and has been once complained of, as a nuisance, to the grand jury." Additional structures for the quarantining of sick inmates were added over the next two decades. (Courtesy of Harvard Art Museums/Fogg Museum, Transfer from the Carpenter Center for the Visual Arts, Social Museum Collection.)

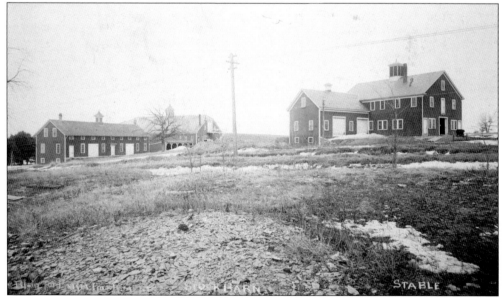

Further accommodations under the leadership of Superintendent Marsh included updates to the slaughterhouse and the addition of a large meat refrigerator so that the meat of any animals slaughtered could be preserved for days, if not weeks, at a time. Farm provisions were seen as essential in providing for the ever-expanding campus. (Courtesy of Harvard Art Museums/Fogg Museum, Transfer from the Carpenter Center for the Visual Arts, Social Museum Collection.)

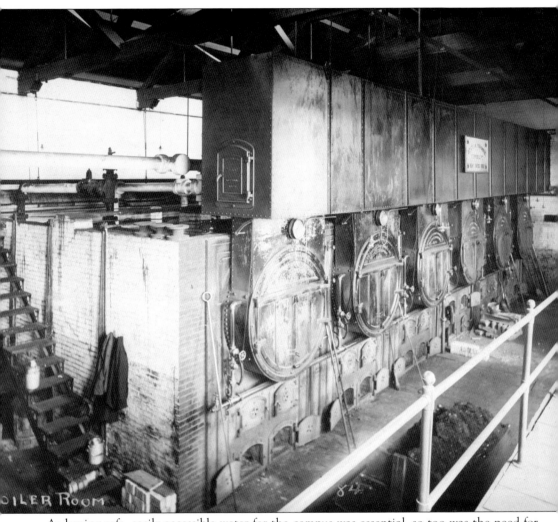

OILER ROOM

As having safe, easily accessible water for the campus was essential, so too was the need for an efficient heating system. The New England winters necessitated heat for the almshouse structures. The administration decided that steam was the best, cheapest, and by far safest mode yet discovered. Although it was among the safest choices at the time, the steam heating apparatus still posed potential danger. Calamity struck the State Almshouse at Tewksbury on October 14, 1862, when one of the steam boilers exploded in the basement of the cookery. One side of the building, as well as part of one end, were blown out, causing extensive damage. The most damage was sustained to the laundry area, where many female patients were completing their daily work when the explosion took place. Five people died instantly, with 20 additional inmates and staff later dying from injuries sustained during the incident. (Courtesy of Harvard Art Museums/Fogg Museum, Transfer from the Carpenter Center for the Visual Arts, Social Museum Collection.)

The explosion of 1862 led to continued improvements to the almshouse's steam-heating system during Superintendent Marsh's tenure at Tewksbury. In 1863, a detached boiler house was constructed outside of the yard, and new, state-of-the-art tubular boilers were installed. Other safety mechanisms were added including new steam pumps, water indicators, a steam whistle, and various gauges. (Courtesy of Harvard Art Museums/Fogg Museum, Transfer from the Carpenter Center for the Visual Arts, Social Museum Collection.)

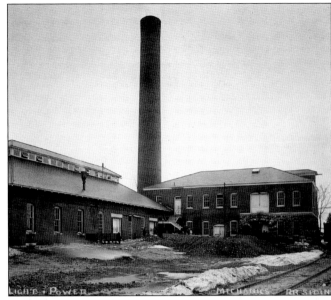

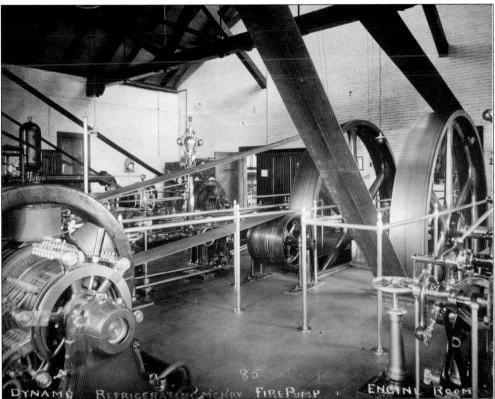

Funds for a new boiler house were appropriated in 1896 to replace the previous one constructed in 1863. The new structure included three new boilers, Corliss steam engines, and a dynamo machine, a generator that provided electricity for the campus. A fire pump was added to the engine room for additional safety in 1903. (Courtesy of Harvard Art Museums/Fogg Museum, Transfer from the Carpenter Center for the Visual Arts, Social Museum Collection.)

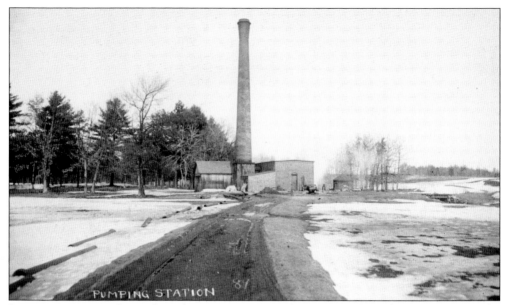

Improvements were also made to the pumping station that provided both drinking water for the residents and water for the steam system. Like the rest of the institution's utilities, the pumping station was coal powered and required boiler system upgrades to improve the safety and efficiency of its production. An entirely new boiler and chimney were installed at the pumping station in 1895. (Courtesy of Harvard Art Museums/Fogg Museum, Transfer from the Carpenter Center for the Visual Arts, Social Museum Collection.)

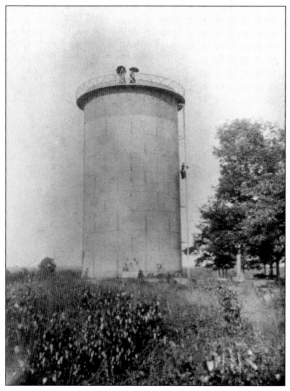

Work on the master reservoir commenced in 1868, and by 1875, about half of the basin had been constructed. In the Annual Report of 1879, Superintendent Marsh noted that this reservoir was capable of storing one million gallons of clear and excellent water. An additional reservoir was added the same year that could hold another million gallons.

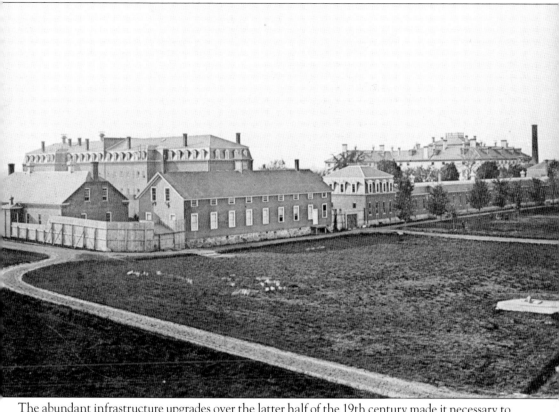

The abundant infrastructure upgrades over the latter half of the 19th century made it necessary to employ a large workforce to sustain the innovations introduced to the institution. The Tewksbury almshouse administrators relied partly on patient labor to maintain both the agricultural and industrial sectors of the almshouse. If a patient was deemed able to work by their class, they were expected to help. The Annual Report of 1883 outlines the three main classes of patients: "—the sick, those in the hospital,—the feeble and deformed, not requiring hospital treatment, yet unable to work,—and the well." Due to various changes in the patient population between 1854 and the 1870s, the "well" were often in short supply. The commonwealth was compelled to invest in adequate medical care for the sick and insane paupers who needed it most, while also maintaining the expanding infrastructure. (Courtesy of the State Library of Massachusetts.)

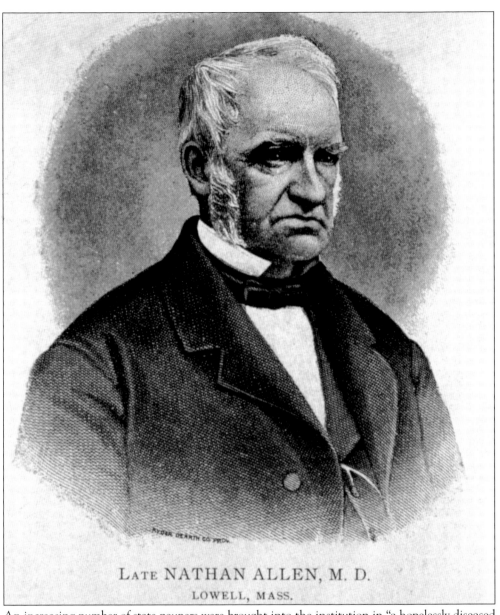

LATE NATHAN ALLEN, M. D.

LOWELL, MASS.

An increasing number of state paupers were brought into the institution in "a hopelessly diseased condition, many of them in fact just ready to perish," in the words of the Annual Report of 1870, necessitating Superintendent Marsh to hire a consulting physician to provide additional support for the medical department in 1870. Dr. Nathan Allen of Lowell, Massachusetts, was an ideal choice as he served on the Massachusetts State Board of Charities and the Lowell Board of Health and was a fierce advocate of institutional reform to ensure the humane treatment of the mentally ill. In the Annual Report of 1870, the medical department called out the town authorities who were transferring extremely sick poor to the almshouse, as it not only violated the law, but also "common humanity demands that the final event, inevitable though it may be, in the case of those whose sands of life have almost run out, should not be hastened by rudely jostling their hour-glass of life by such removal." The increasing number of sick inmates led to an expanding death rate that only continued to rise toward the end of the 19th century. (Courtesy of the US National Library of Medicine.)

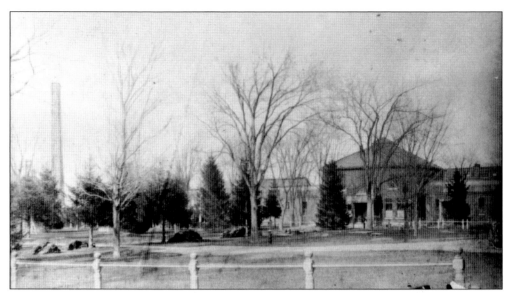

With the increasingly sick population of incoming paupers, almshouse administrators pleaded with the legislature for funding to construct a new hospital building. In 1870, an appropriation of $20,000 was allocated to cover the costs of erection, equipment, and heating of the new hospital, which was designed to accommodate 160 patients.

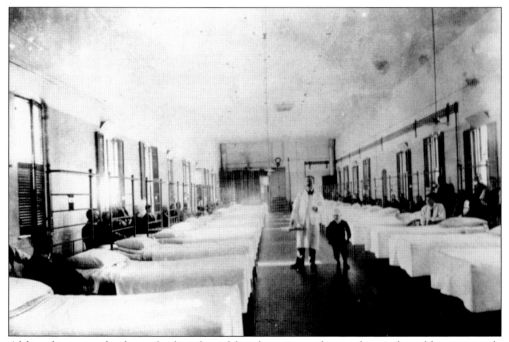

Although supposed to house both male and female patients, the new hospital would come to only serve sick male paupers. From its opening, there were concerns regarding the ventilation system, and further funds were needed to improve the airflow. An additional improvement came in 1874 when water closets were installed to replace the previous earth closets.

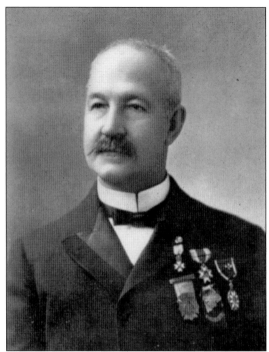

Medical assistance in caring for the almshouse's progressively sicker residents was provided by local physicians. Around the fall of 1874, Dr. Moses Greeley Parker of Lowell began visiting the hospital to voluntarily perform any operation "on the eye or ear, or any other intricate surgery that might be required." This ushered in new medical offerings, as prior surgical procedures were limited in scope. (Courtesy of the Dracut Historical Society.)

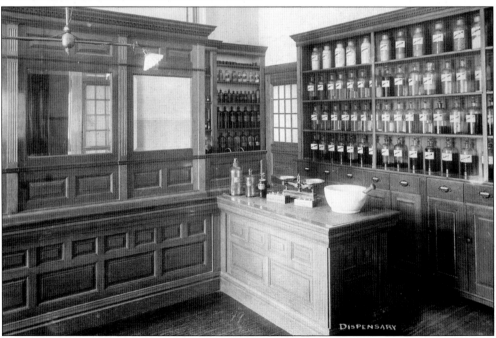

Other improvements came to the medical department including the transition to the metric system of weights and measurements for dispensing medicine to patients in the hospital and asylum. William H. Lathrop, primary physician at the almshouse after the retirement of Dr. J.D. Nichols in 1875, saw this change as a great gain to allow for both increased customization in drug concoction and minimizing possible mistakes in dosage. (Courtesy of Harvard Art Museums/Fogg Museum, Transfer from the Carpenter Center for the Visual Arts, Social Museum Collection.)

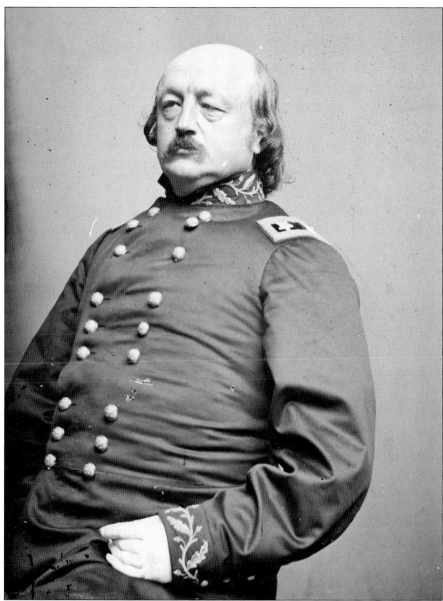

Although improvements were made to almshouse medical care in the 1870s and 1880s, Superintendent Marsh repeatedly came under fire for the high mortality rate exhibited year after year. The sanitary conditions were called into question in 1874, which was the beginning of the end for Marsh's tenure. Enter Benjamin Butler, a rugged and controversial politician who had served as a general in the Union army during the Civil War, and became governor of Massachusetts in January 1883. In his inaugural address, he issued a scathing charge against the administrators of the Tewksbury almshouse for gross misconduct and unsanitary conditions. A full investigation was launched, with the State Board of Health, Lunacy, and Charity taking control of the almshouse as Governor Butler suspended the institution's trustees from carrying out their duties as of April 28, 1883. The investigative committee spent several months in the spring and summer of 1883 visiting the almshouse, hearing testimony, and examining evidence of mismanagement. (Courtesy of the Prints and Photographs Division of the Library of Congress.)

Among the allegations was the claim from Governor Butler that hundreds of deceased infants and adults were sold to medical institutions in Boston. The investigative committee found that some bodies were sold for anatomical research, but it was done fully within the law. Butler continued to insist on wrongdoing, going as far as to claim that bodies were sent away to be tanned and used for leatherwork. (Courtesy of Harvard Medical Library in the Francis A. Countway Library of Medicine.)

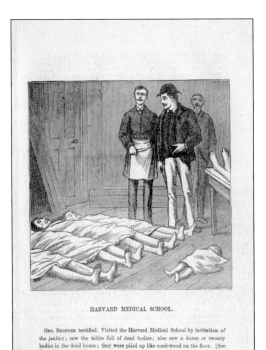

HARVARD MEDICAL SCHOOL.

Geo. Skinner testified: Visited the Harvard Medical School by invitation of the janitor; saw the tables full of dead bodies; also saw a dozen or twenty bodies in the dead house; they were piled up like cord-wood on the floor. [See Record, page 3,017.]

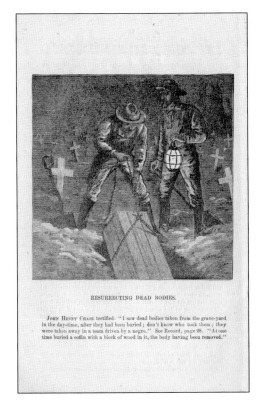

RESURRECTING DEAD BODIES.

John Henry Chase testified: "I saw dead bodies taken from the grave-yard in the day-time, after they had been buried; don't know who took them; they were taken away in a team driven by a negro." See Record, page 28. "At one time buried a coffin with a block of wood in it, the body having been removed."

Another assertion by Governor Butler was that after a deceased patient was buried in the almshouse cemetery, they would be dug up and sold off to a medical school for profit. He also professed that "in more instances than one, funeral services were held over supposed remains," claiming that coffins were filled with wood to deceive the patients' loved ones. (Courtesy of Harvard Medical Library in the Francis A. Countway Library of Medicine.)

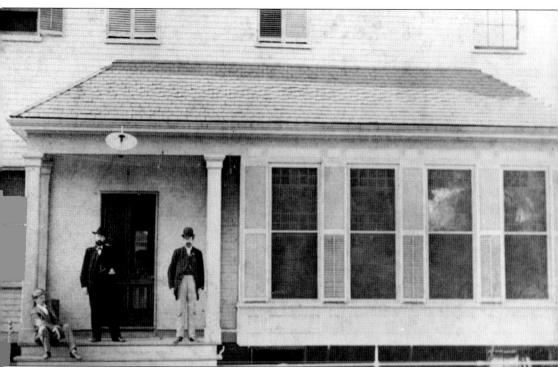

Despite Governor Butler's persistence and the accounts presented by individuals who alleged administrative negligence, the investigative committee ultimately found the main charges of the governor against the State Almshouse at Tewksbury and its administrators "groundless and cruel." Instead of appearing admirable, Governor Butler was labeled an embarrassment, having needlessly brought shame and humiliation upon the commonwealth. The committee did identify some carelessness by members of the almshouse administration and trustees, but nothing that substantiated removal from office. Instead, the committee requested better bookkeeping and review of policies, especially in regard to nepotism, as several members of the Marsh family were employed at the almshouse. Ultimately, Thomas J. Marsh, Nancy F. Marsh, and Thomas J. Marsh Jr. all resigned from their service to the State Almshouse at Tewksbury in 1883. The only member of the Marsh family to remain was Charles B. Marsh (left), who served as clerk. Chester Irving Fisher (center) assumed the role of superintendent and resident physician, and John H. Cocker (right) became the assistant superintendent.

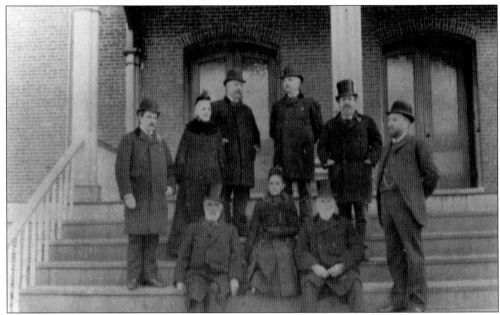

The years following the 1883 investigation saw continued development of the institution's hospital functions as it chiefly served the sick poor of the commonwealth. The new superintendent, C. Irving Fisher, stressed the importance of additional hospital accommodations in terms of both physical space and number of staff. The newly appointed board of trustees, who took over governance of the almshouse in 1884, also emphasized the need for overall improvements to the institution, citing poor funding from the legislature for far too long. Clara T. Leonard, a member of the board of trustees, expressed her discontent with the commonwealth that such a "rich and prosperous State, year after year, cries out, 'Cut down pauper expense,' " while the current per capita appropriation was already too meager to provide adequate care for the paupers of the state.

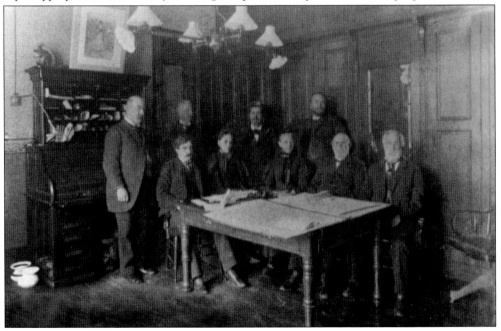

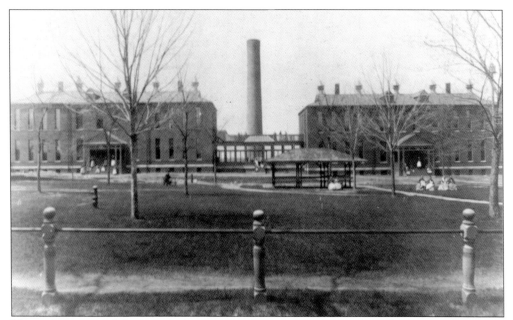

Upon the urging of the board of trustees and Superintendent Fisher, the legislature in 1886 approved the disbursement of $75,000 for the construction of a new hospital for female patients to replace the old workshops and storehouse buildings that previously served as accommodations for female sick paupers. The new hospital consisted of two rectangular two-story brick buildings connected by a sunroom.

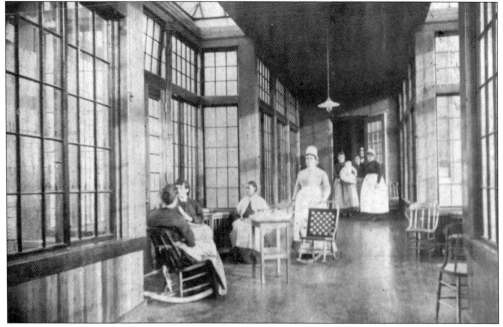

The Female Hospital opened on January 6, 1888, with a capacity of 200 patients, 100 in each wing. At the time, it was considered among the most magnificent hospitals in the United States, offering the most economical and efficient ventilating systems of any hospital of its size, with every sanitary convenience available, as well as a designated operating room for women.

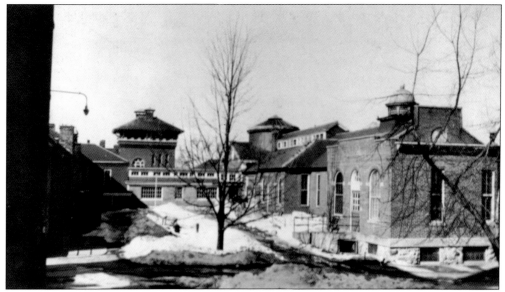

Unlike the new Female Hospital, the hospital accommodations for male patients by the late 1880s were abysmal. The Male Hospital lacked proper ventilation and suffered from overcrowding due to its insufficient size. After repeated requests to the governor, the legislature of 1889 allocated $35,000 for the construction of a new hospital that would connect to the existing structure.

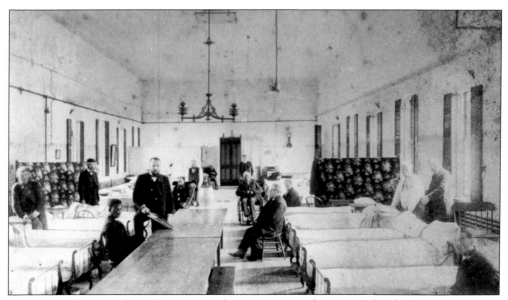

The new Male Hospital ward was occupied in June 1890 and accommodated up to 50 patients in a confined environment. The ward was mostly utilized for acute patients, as well as those with more contagious diseases. During the same year, renovations were made to the existing hospital including a new dispensary, library, and operating room.

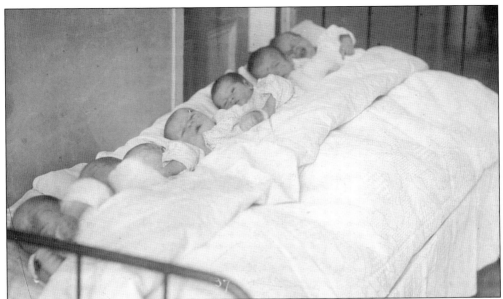

The maternity department also received improvements in the 1880s and 1890s after several decades of a high confinement and mortality rate among infants. Babies could end up at the almshouse for several reasons: the infant could have been abandoned by their mother, sent to the almshouse through some friend or suspected goodwilled individual, or left behind when their patient mother escaped the facility. (Courtesy of Harvard Art Museums/Fogg Museum, Transfer from the Carpenter Center for the Visual Arts, Social Museum Collection.)

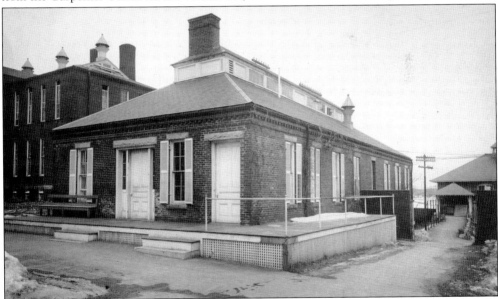

Mothers and infants were put up in the makeshift Maternity Hospital before extensive renovations were completed in 1888 and 1899 to improve sanitation and the overall comfort and convenience of nurses and patients alike. Almshouse administrators hoped that the improved conditions would help reduce the high mortality rate that plagued the institution due to the often feeble state of infants in their care. (Courtesy of Harvard Art Museums/Fogg Museum, Transfer from the Carpenter Center for the Visual Arts, Social Museum Collection.)

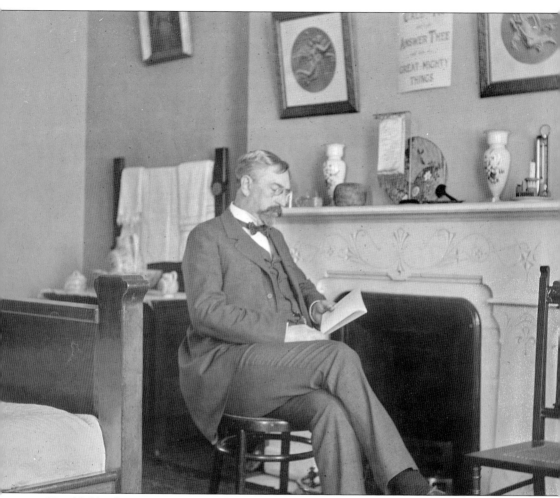

Heralded by the trustees as a confident, faithful, and efficient officer, Superintendent Fisher had many accomplishments during his eight years of service to the State Almshouse at Tewksbury. He refined the classification of patients while applying business methods consistent with hospital requirements to improve overall almshouse administration. He established a consulting board made up of revered Boston physicians to provide advice and support for the betterment of the hospital department. And he initiated an intern program in conjunction with Harvard Medical School, among other accolades. The superintendency of Dr. Fisher brought the almshouse into a new and prosperous era and set the stage for further medical success under Fisher's successor, Dr. Herbert Howard. (Digital positive from the original gelatin silver negative in the George Eastman Museum's collection.)

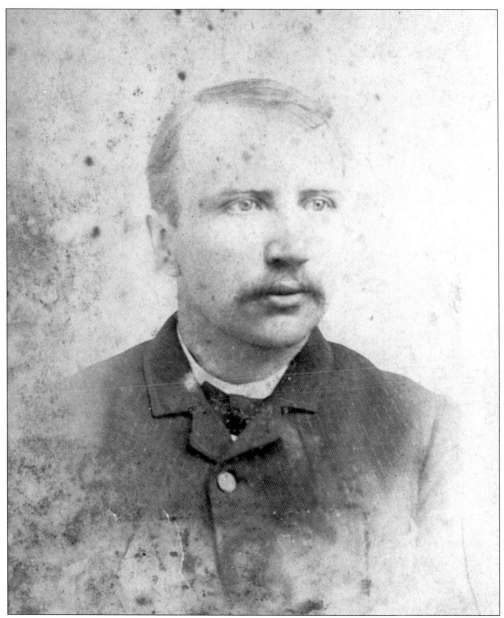

Herbert Burr Howard completed his medical studies at Harvard University in 1884 and served as a physician at Tewksbury before being promoted to superintendent. His approach to the superintendent role was to build on many of the hospital advances that his predecessor made, including continuing the internship program with Harvard Medical School. Howard also supported additional training opportunities for staff, especially nurses, and succeeded in infrastructure improvements for the campus. Howard served the State Almshouse until 1897, before being appointed to the position of resident physician at Massachusetts General Hospital. He also served on the State Board of Insanity and as president of the American Hospital Association, and became the first superintendent of the Peter Bent Brigham Hospital before his retirement.

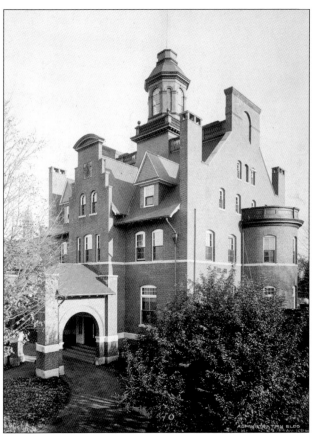

As the hospital campus continued to expand, the original almshouse building was showing its age. And being made out of wood, it posed a constant safety hazard. Consequently, from 1894 to 1895, the new Administration Building was constructed in front of the old building. After construction was complete, the old wooden structure was torn down, and the yard was enclosed around the new building. Outside the stone wall was the new Superintendent's Home, providing living quarters for Dr. Howard and his family. These buildings, along with the new Women's Dormitory extension, were designed by architect John A. Fox and completed by L.E. Locke of Lawrence, Massachusetts. (Courtesy of Harvard Art Museums/Fogg Museum, Transfer from the Carpenter Center for the Visual Arts, Social Museum Collection.)

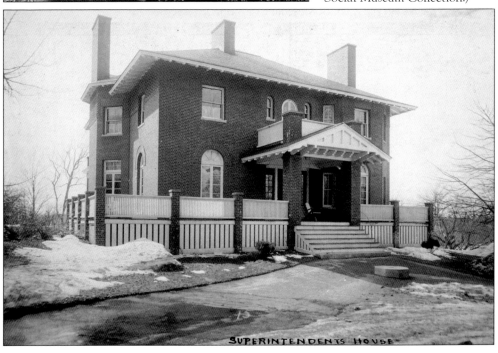

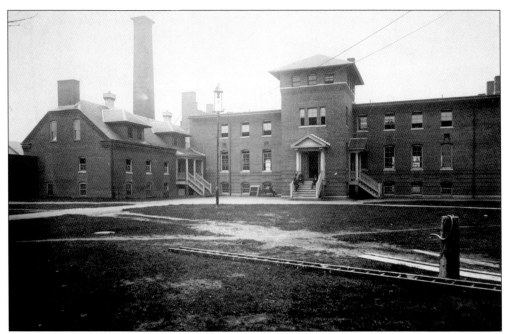

The original cookery next to the wooden almshouse structure was also becoming outdated. After the 1862 explosion, numerous renovations, and advancements in cooking machinery, it was apparent that the institution needed a new, more centralized kitchen for its growing campus. A new kitchen was situated at the south end of the yard, with a dining hall built alongside it. The dining hall allowed up to 900 patients to eat at one time and was used by patients in the almshouse and insane departments. An industrial refrigerator and pork cellar were also added in 1894. (Both, courtesy of Harvard Art Museums/Fogg Museum, Transfer from the Carpenter Center for the Visual Arts, Social Museum Collection.)

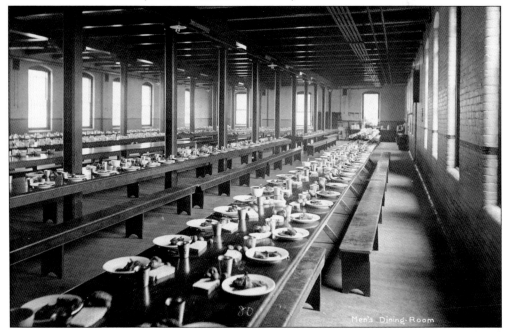

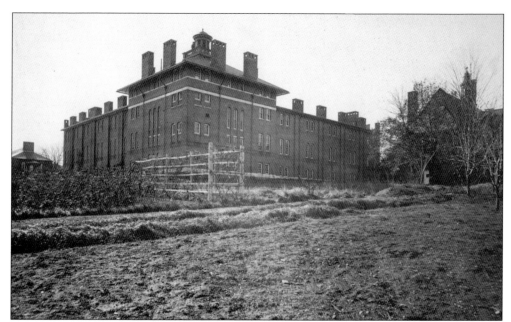

There was also a need for increased dormitory space for the male population. This structure was completed in 1894, but an expansion was added in 1900. The new wing of the Men's Dormitory included a smoking room, sanitary section, fireproof staircase, and officer's room. (Courtesy of Harvard Art Museums/Fogg Museum, Transfer from the Carpenter Center for the Visual Arts, Social Museum Collection.)

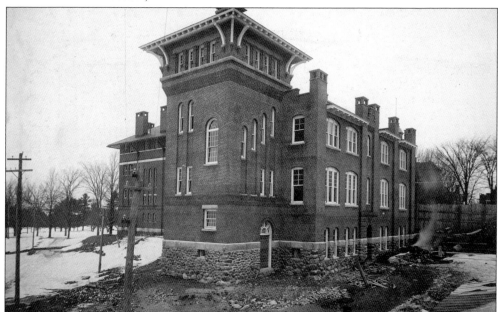

Opened around February 1, 1895, the Women's Dormitory was similar in appearance to the Men's Dormitory, but on the western side of campus. It too received an expansion, with the first floor providing additional resident beds and a sitting room for aged women and the second floor providing dormitory space for children and a dayroom. (Courtesy of Harvard Art Museums/Fogg Museum, Transfer from the Carpenter Center for the Visual Arts, Social Museum Collection.)

When the former chapel was converted to the Men's Asylum during the winter of 1883–1884, the campus lacked a sufficient location for religious services. For almost 10 years, chaplains were forced to hold services in one of the dayrooms in the asylum for insane women. These rooms were far too small for the congregants and posed safety concerns for having a large number of sick or insane patients in a confined space. In 1896, after years of requesting an allocation from the state, the construction of a chapel was commissioned that could hold up to 500 patients. The project was completed in 1898 for a total cost of $12,000. (Both, courtesy of Harvard Art Museums/Fogg Museum, Transfer from the Carpenter Center for the Visual Arts, Social Museum Collection.)

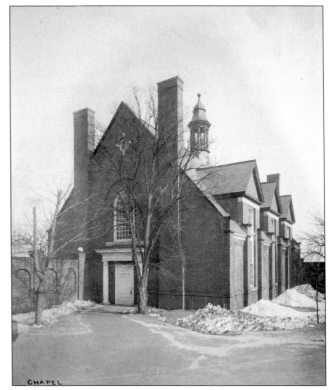

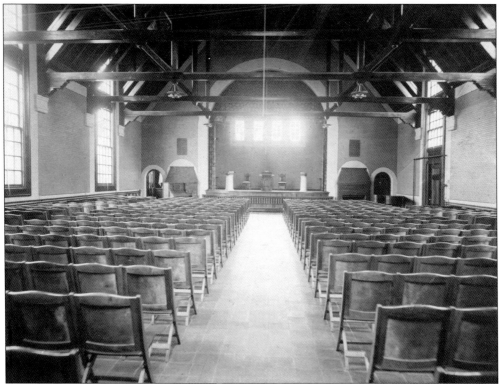

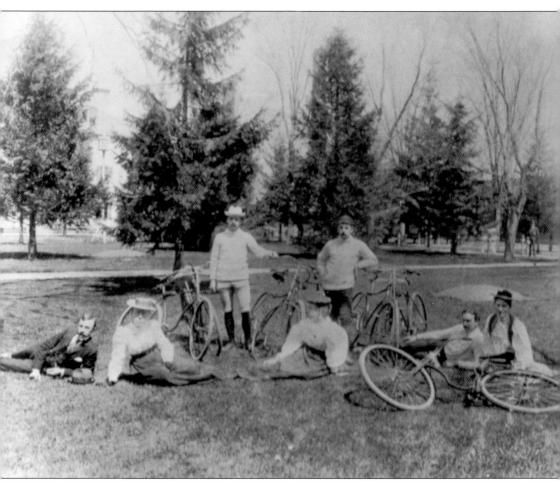

The accomplishments of Dr. Herbert B. Howard were plentiful, but his time as superintendent came to an end in May 1897. He left the almshouse in the capable hands of his apprentice, Dr. John Holyoke Nichols (third from left). Born in Danvers, Nichols went on to study at Harvard and completed an internship at the State Almshouse at Tewksbury as part of his senior year. He worked in private practice for one year before being appointed assistant physician at Tewksbury. In 1896, he was promoted to assistant superintendent, and upon Dr. Howard's resignation, Nichols was appointed superintendent in 1897. Although his predecessors were adept in hospital management and care of state paupers, the greatest progress was to come with Dr. Nichols as the head of what would become the Tewksbury State Hospital.

Two

Caring for the Insane

Between 1845 and 1860, the United States experienced a massive influx of immigrants from Northern Europe who were seeking refuge from war and famine. Massachusetts received many immigrants who came from Ireland and had strong ties to Catholicism, which was concerning to the Anglo-Protestant majority in New England at the time. Anti-immigrant rhetoric influenced mental health policies throughout the 19th and 20th centuries, as leading psychiatrists and medical practitioners improperly associated nativity and social class with prevalence of insanity. As a consequence, immigrants had a higher probability of being diagnosed as insane.

Although the State Almshouse at Tewksbury was not specifically intended to support the mentally ill from the outset, it quickly became a receptacle "for a certain class of the insane paupers, such as are demented and harmlessly insane, who are regarded as incurables, and who mainly need kind treatment and a home," as noted in the Annual Report of 1856. It was thought that this class of patients could be cared for in the state almshouses far more inexpensively than within the lunatic hospitals since these "incurables" were not receiving active treatment for their conditions. The State Almshouse at Tewksbury started accepting transfers from Worcester Insane Hospital and Taunton Insane Hospital right away, the beginning of a long history serving the mentally ill of Massachusetts.

With the formal establishment of an insane department, the almshouse needed to provide boarding for this new type of patient. The administration utilized remaining appropriations from 1855 to convert an outbuilding into wards for the insane to keep them separated from the state paupers in the almshouse department. These patients quickly outgrew the small wooden building fitted up for their care, and requests were made several years in a row to provide suitable accommodations for their growing numbers, but it was not until 1866 that relief came.

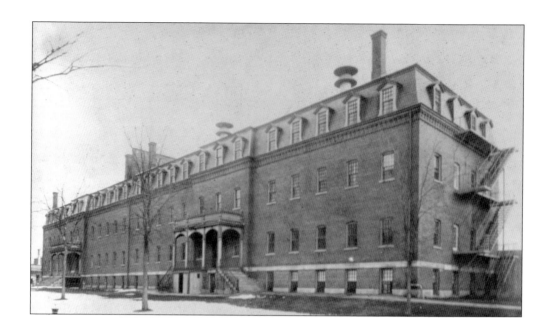

The year 1866 brought the construction of the first substantial structure for the mentally ill at the State Almshouse at Tewksbury. Built to accommodate 100 harmless insane, the Long Asylum welcomed 40 females and about 40 males during the summer of 1866 upon its opening. The cost for the new asylum was $33,500, but it was suspected that it would be a cost savings to the state to house the "harmless insane" at the almshouse instead of the lunatic hospitals, which were costlier to maintain. The almshouse administrators also benefited from the exchange, as this category of insane proved to be useful laborers on the farm and in the various trade shops.

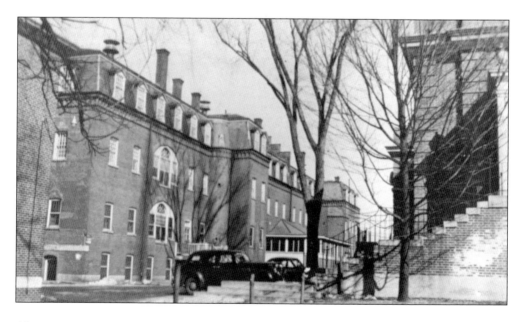

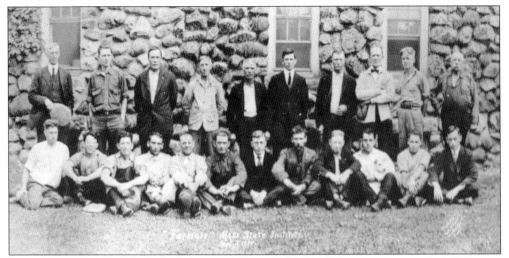

William Tuke's theory on moral treatment for the mentally ill and the mission of social rehabilitation were instituted early on by the Tewksbury administration. Those labeled as the "harmless insane" in the mid-19th century were mostly assigned to agricultural work, as "tilling of the soil must continue to be our chief employment," as stated in the Annual Report of 1866, as it "may yet become a source of considerable profit in ready cash" for the almshouse. Cultivation of the land remained the primary focus for patient labor in pursuit of institutional self-sufficiency well into the 20th century.

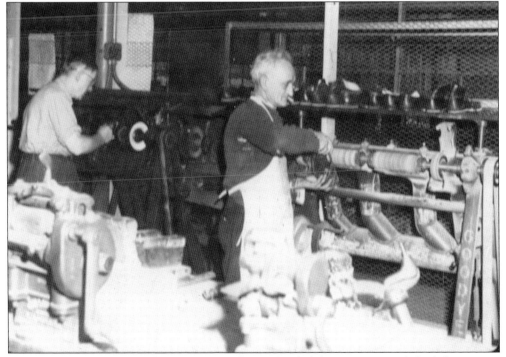

Aside from the benefit to the institution, the work rehabilitation approach had therapeutic value for patients as well as providing specialized training that would enable them to become self-sufficient once they returned to the workforce. The shoe shop, paint shop, glass shop, repair shop, and storehouse all conscripted patients, primarily males, to carry out routine duties.

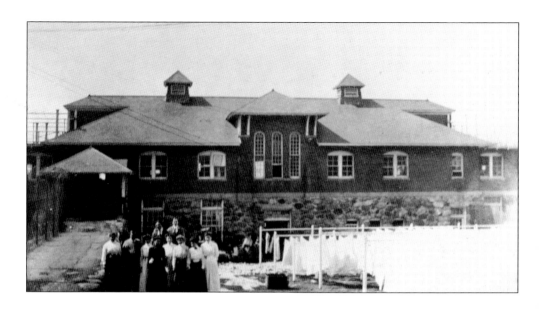

Female patients of the insane department were chosen to carry out the domestic work of the institution, and many worked in the laundry in various capacities. Some women were employed to knit blankets and bedding, some to mend clothes, some to make up beds with fresh linens, and some to visit the various wards to retrieve and deliver the laundered items. Later, with the opening of a new laundry building in 1901, capacity expanded, allowing women in both the almshouse and insane departments to contribute to the overall output of products manufactured on-site. Between October 1, 1900, and October 1, 1901, the house department made 27,941 articles and the insane department made 29,353 articles of items ranging from crib sheets to burial robes.

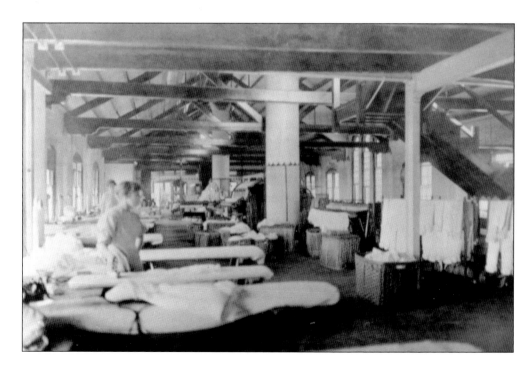

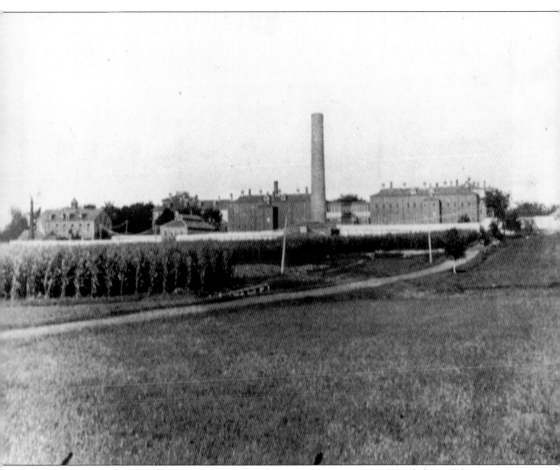

The implementation of work therapy as a form of restorative treatment at Tewksbury did not come without concern or criticism from other members of the medical profession at the time. Several leading psychiatrists and mental hospital superintendents in New England did not believe that the work therapy program was particularly beneficial in helping patients recover, nor did they feel that it would be economically beneficial enough to the institution to warrant its continuation. Yet Superintendent Marsh spoke most boisterously of its effectiveness, saying that the thoughts of an insane patient "must in some way be turned from brooding over his own ills, and transferred from the objects his own imaginings have created to the realities of the world from which they have long been isolated" and that "employment of the physical powers in manual labor is one of the essentials" toward the goal of restoring the mentally ill to their right mind. It also proved to be financially beneficial for the Commonwealth of Massachusetts, leading to a steady influx of those deemed insane to the almshouse.

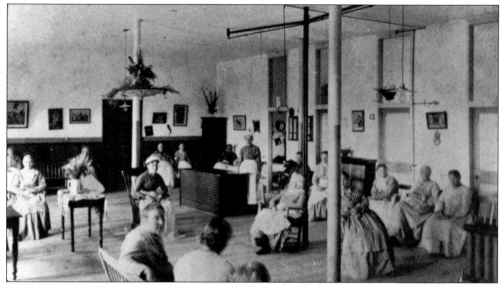

As more patients were transferred from the lunatic hospitals to Tewksbury, further accommodations were needed. An appropriation was made for $25,000 in the winter of 1870 to expand the Long Asylum for an additional 150 patients. The expansion was completed entirely by patient labor, except for one officer and a hired hand, and became occupied in December 1872.

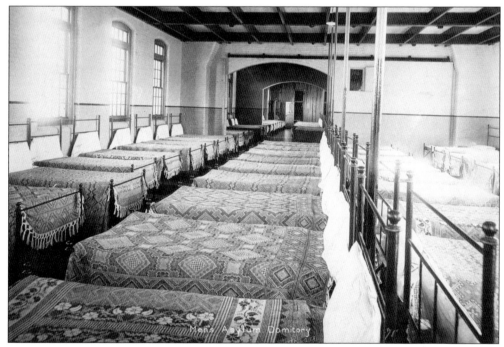

The addition quickly proved nonviable as patients outnumbered available beds. Appointed physician for the insane in 1874, Dr. James M. Whitaker noted that as of October 1 of that year, there were 319 patients and only 291 beds in the Long Asylum. He proposed sweeping changes to the organization of the insane department. (Courtesy of Harvard Art Museums/Fogg Museum, Transfer from the Carpenter Center for the Visual Arts, Social Museum Collection.)

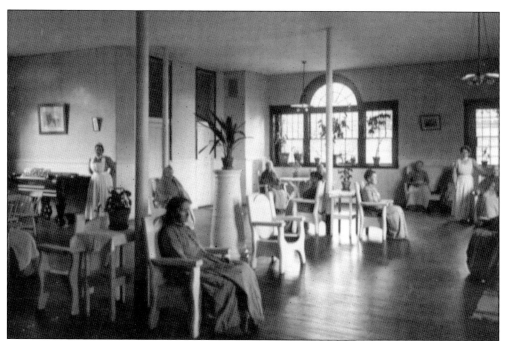

Due to overcrowding in the Long Asylum, there were regularly 60 to 75 patients in a room no larger than 40 by 50 feet. Whitaker sought to remedy these cramped quarters by remodeling the structure in order to "render the dreary journey of life less dreary" for insane patients. The goal was to have no more than 25 patients in one room at the same time in hopes of improving their classification and both mental and physical health, which in turn would contribute to an enhancement in their overall wellbeing. Grouping patients based on mental cognition also made it possible to offer better treatment for those who could benefit from medical intervention.

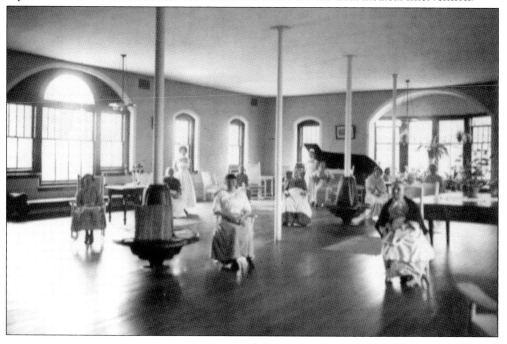

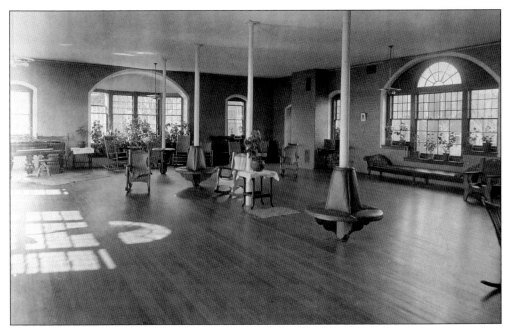

Dr. Whitaker also recommended cosmetic upgrades to the asylum building to improve patient morale. He suggested that each sitting-room be outfitted with a reading table stacked with books or newspapers and games, such as backgammon, checkers, or cards, to provide amusement to patients. The dayrooms were adorned with potted plants meant to bring fresh air and a sense of calm to patients, and pianos were added for the musically inclined. The walls were decorated with plates and prints of suitable character. This work was undertaken with the goal of providing the patients with "objects of interest and beauty to cheer the loneliness of their long hours of pain and suffering." (Both, courtesy of Harvard Art Museums/Fogg Museum, Transfer from the Carpenter Center for the Visual Arts, Social Museum Collection.)

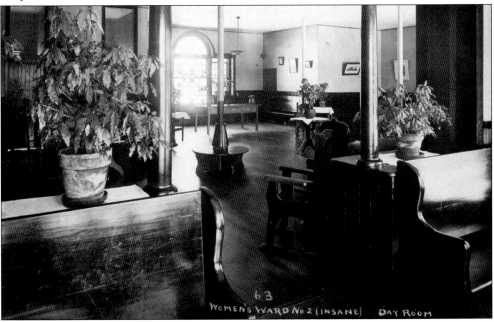

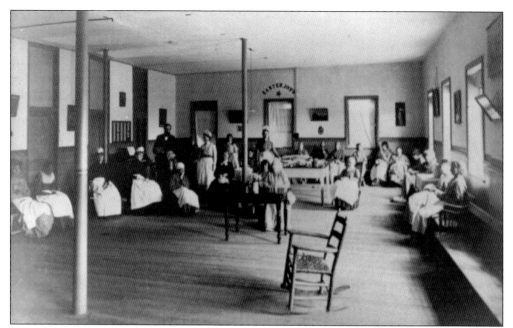

In 1874, Long Asylum received additional upgrades, including partitioning each hall into single rooms for patients. This not only provided more comfort to patients, a constant goal of the almshouse administration, but also provided seclusion in case a mentally ill patient became violent.

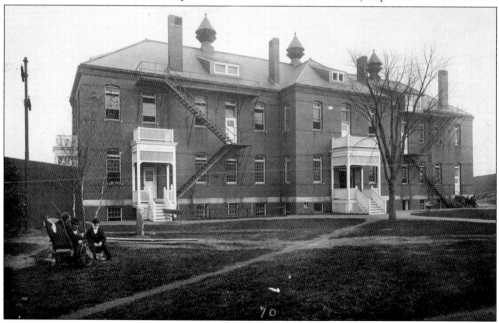

From the late 1870s to 1886, the insane department remained at a status quo, with the majority of patients being female. That changed in 1886 when 43 male insane patients were admitted to Tewksbury and put up in makeshift quarters in the old wooden chapel building. After years of requests, an appropriation was made for $20,000 in 1891 for the construction of a new asylum for men, Asylum No. 4. (Courtesy of Harvard Art Museums/Fogg Museum, Transfer from the Carpenter Center for the Visual Arts, Social Museum Collection.)

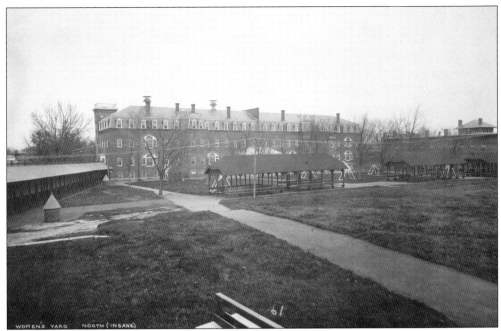

The legislature of 1891 also approved funds for the building of new summerhouses in the female insane yard. The new summerhouses featured concrete floors and were built to be more spacious to accommodate the growing number of female patients admitted to the department. (Courtesy of Harvard Art Museums/Fogg Museum, Transfer from the Carpenter Center for the Visual Arts, Social Museum Collection.)

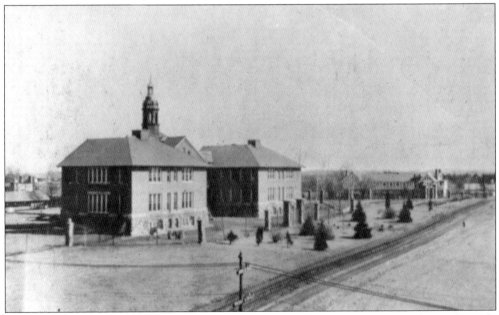

The yards were altered and expanded many times throughout the late 1800s and into the early 1900s. Men were separated from women, children separated from adults, and the sane separated from those deemed insane. The goal of the extensive green space was restorative treatment in providing the opportunity for ample fresh air and natural light for patients.

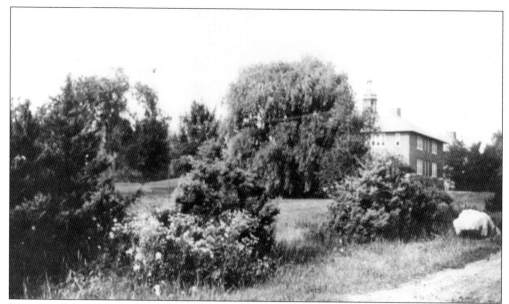

Trees, shrubs, and flowers were planted to add beauty and tranquility to the yards. Along with a staff gardener, patients worked to maintain the landscape and continually improve it, with the incorporation of more concrete paths that had untold value for the patients who walked them.

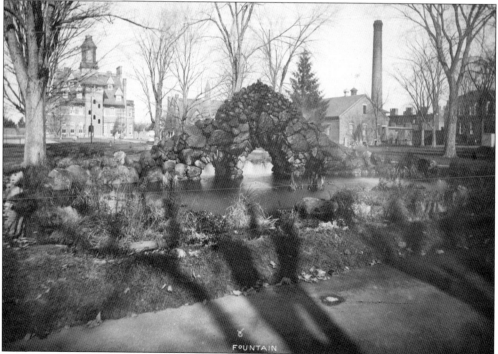

A fountain was added in 1895 to the center of the yard where the old greenhouse once stood to serve as an ornamental landscape feature. The rustic fountain was built around a small pond with stones excavated from the growing farm. The labor was supplied by Dr. Nichols, assistant physician, who would become superintendent in 1897. (Courtesy of Harvard Art Museums/Fogg Museum, Transfer from the Carpenter Center for the Visual Arts, Social Museum Collection.)

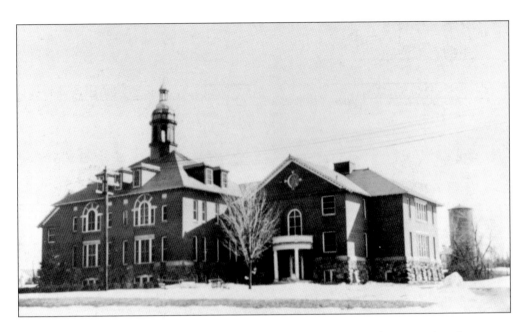

In his last act as superintendent, Dr. Howard witnessed the opening of a new asylum for women at the southern edge of the yard. Opened on May 1, 1897, and designed by John A. Fox, the new asylum was reserved for violent female cases in the insane department. Asylum No. 8, or the Belcher Insane Hospital, was named after J. White Belcher, longtime chairman of the Board of Trustees of the State Almshouse at Tewksbury. Belcher became acquainted with the almshouse in 1874 in his work as inspector of the State Farm at Bridgewater, then overseeing the State Almshouse at Tewksbury, and finally in his appointment to the board of trustees at its establishment in 1884. He served as chairman from 1884 until his death on February 9, 1906.

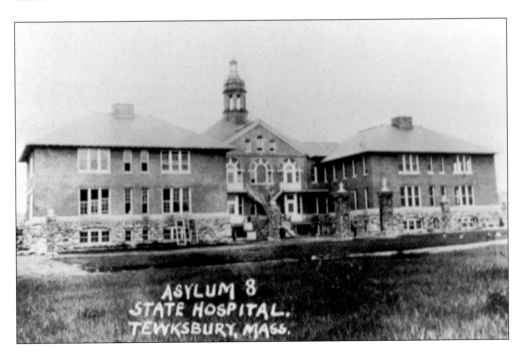

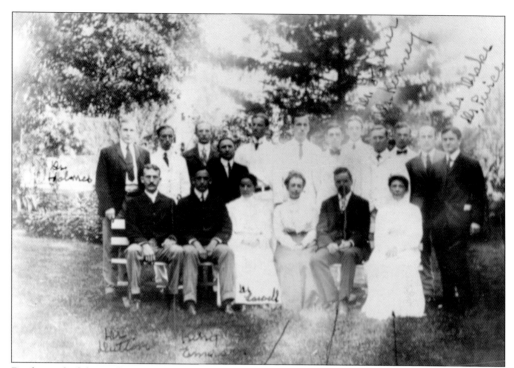

By the end of the 19th century, the State Almshouse at Tewksbury served a significant role in the care of the mentally ill. The insane department averaged about 500 residents, which necessitated reevaluation of the categorization of patients. The administration of 1898 saw nearly all forms and stages of mental disease and classified the insane into six different groups. The insane were beginning to make up a larger percentage of the patient population.

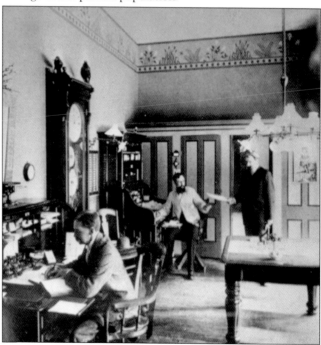

Categorization and organization went hand-in-hand in providing for the structured environment essential to the care of the mentally ill. In 1886, a Howard electric clock was installed in the almshouse office with wires connecting to every department. Originally used to ensure night watchmen were performing their duties, it eventually served to regulate daily activities in the wards.

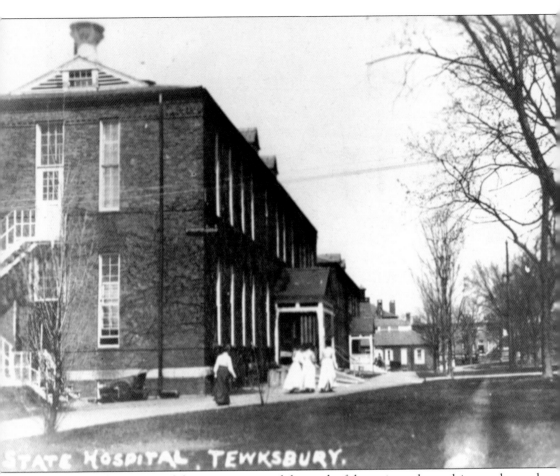

STATE HOSPITAL, TEWKSBURY.

As the almshouse entered the next century and the needs of the patients changed, it was advanced by the new superintendent, Dr. John H. Nichols, that a name change was necessary to reflect the conditions and workings of the institution. By act of the legislature, the name was officially changed from the State Almshouse to the State Hospital on May 23, 1900. The board of trustees and administrative staff believed that the term "state hospital" was synonymous with the true character of the institution, as the word hospital expressed "happily the relation of the State to the three main classes for whom provision is expressly made; the insane, the sick and the destitute," according to the Annual Report of 1900.

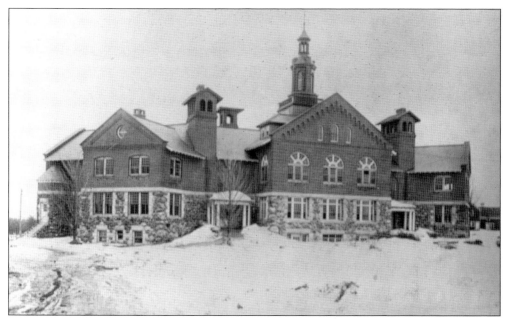

With Dr. Nichols at the helm, a major building campaign took place from the late 1800s into the early 1900s to refurbish older structures and erect new buildings to further the mission of the State Hospital at Tewksbury. Construction on Asylum No. 7 began in 1901. It officially opened its doors in 1904 to house the male insane. Built for $50,000, the asylum was designed in three sections to accommodate various classifications of insanity. Great care was also given in regard to heating and ventilation and to provide for abundant sunshine throughout the building. Asylum No. 7 came to be known as the Hecht Asylum after board of trustees member Jacob H. Hecht. It was later renamed the Anne Sullivan Center to honor one of the almshouse's most famous residents. (Below, courtesy of Harvard Art Museums/Fogg Museum, Transfer from the Carpenter Center for the Visual Arts, Social Museum Collection.)

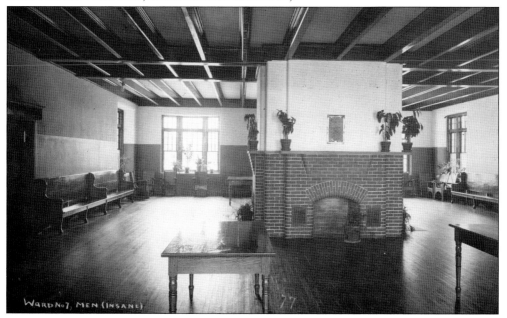

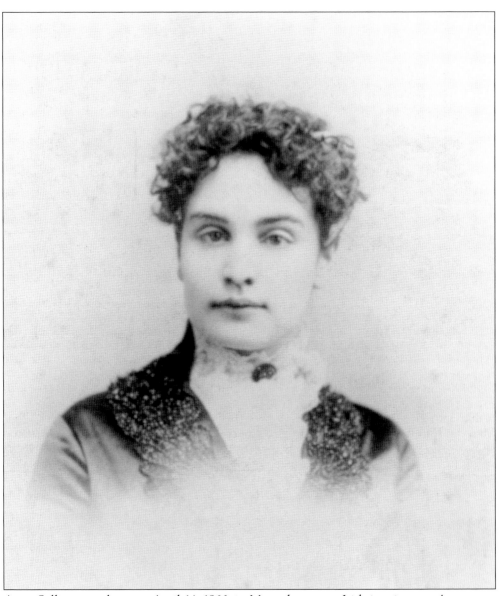

Anne Sullivan was born on April 14, 1866, in Massachusetts to Irish immigrants. At a young age, she developed trachoma, a bacterial infection that affects the eyes, which resulted in visual impairment for the remainder of her life. About two years after the death of their mother, Anne and her brother Jimmie were admitted to the State Almshouse at Tewksbury. Anne was 10 years old at the time. They resided together in the women's ward until May 1876, when Jimmie succumbed to tubercular meningitis. While at Tewksbury, Anne received two unsuccessful eye operations before being sent to the Soeurs de la Charite Hospital in Lowell, Massachusetts, where she underwent another failed eye surgery. After being readmitted to Tewksbury, she convinced the state inspector to allow her transfer to the Perkins School for the Blind. She graduated as valedictorian and underwent a partially successful operation that allowed her to regain some of her vision. Shortly after graduation, Sullivan secured a job as teacher for Helen Keller, the famous author and political activist who was both deaf and blind. (Courtesy of Perkins School for the Blind Archives, Watertown, Massachusetts.)

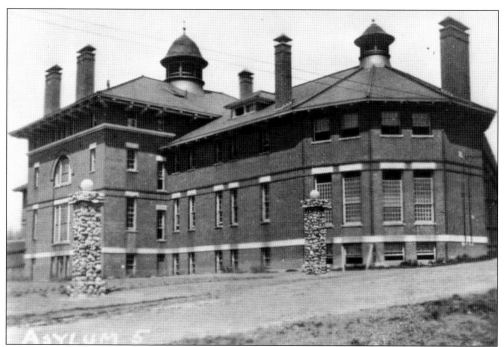

As admissions in the women's insane department continued to grow, the superintendent requested the construction of a new asylum for women in 1901. The work on the structure did not commence until 1904, and progress was slow. It was not until October 1, 1906, that the violent and "excited" female patients moved in. Asylum No. 5, or the Rice Building as it would later be called, was designed with secure rooms to contain dangerous patients. (Below, courtesy of Harvard Art Museums/Fogg Museum, Transfer from the Carpenter Center for the Visual Arts, Social Museum Collection.)

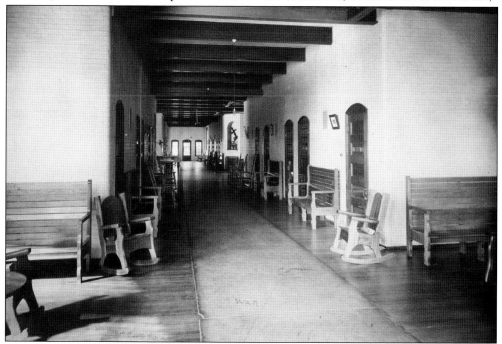

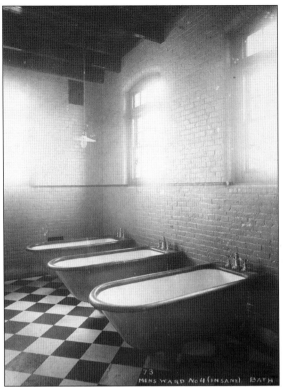

The insane department remained at a status quo for the first half of the 20th century. No additional structures were built; rather; the existing structures received periodic upgrades. Asylum No. 5 and the Belcher Building both benefited from the installation of new tubs with Leonard valves for continuous baths, a form of hydrotherapy, in 1917. (Courtesy of Harvard Art Museums/ Fogg Museum, Transfer from the Carpenter Center for the Visual Arts, Social Museum Collection.)

Patients in the insane department continued to perform general housekeeping, laundry, and kitchen work, as well as work on the farm, stable, and grounds throughout the early 1900s. Making up one third of the population, these patients supplied the majority of the work to keep the institution operational, as the general hospital and convalescent departments were unfit for physical labor.

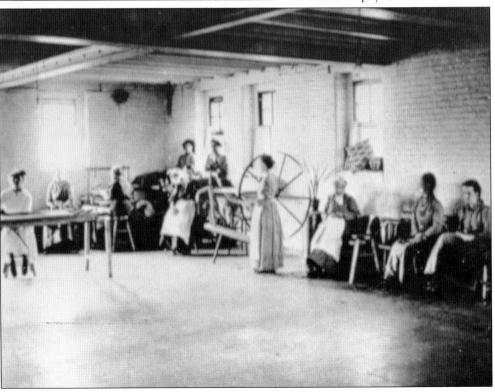

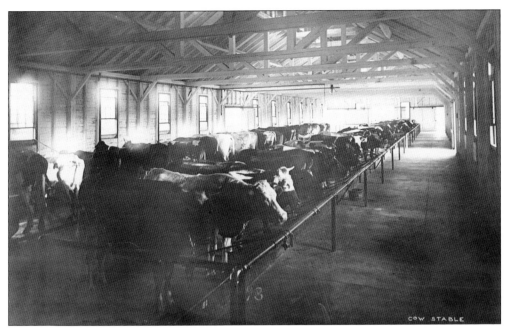

Tewksbury had a plentiful supply of cattle, as the milk was used to supply the sick and infants with nourishment. A new cow stable was added in 1898 for $3,200 and accommodated 82 head of cattle. The structure was built with safety and health in mind, with various forms of egress in case of fire, a floor made of cement, and tie-ups made of iron for enhanced hygiene. It also was constructed with high ceilings to provide ample fresh air for the herd, but unfortunately, disease did strike. When a tuberculin test was administered on the cattle in 1898, many tested positive and were either slaughtered or quarantined. Tuberculosis struck the herd again in 1919, requiring the elimination of all dairy cows at the urging of the Department of Animal Industry. (Both, courtesy of Harvard Art Museums/Fogg Museum, Transfer from the Carpenter Center for the Visual Arts, Social Museum Collection.)

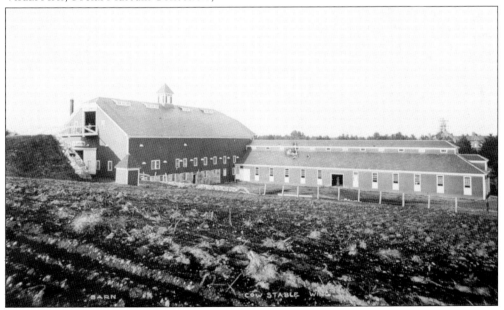

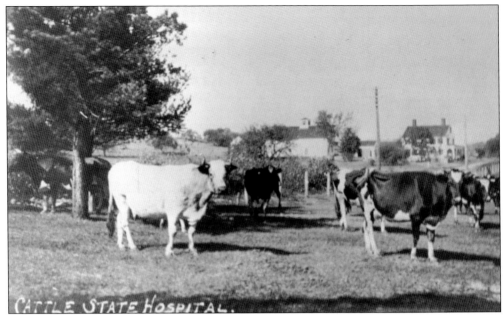

The institution's livestock was plentiful, requiring ever-expanding barn and farm space. In 1890, the livestock at the almshouse were appraised as being worth $9,508.20. That same year, 10,274 pounds of pork, 477 pounds of poultry, and 4,628 pounds of beef was produced on the farm to be used by the institution, in addition to 39,770 gallons of milk and 2,820 dozen eggs.

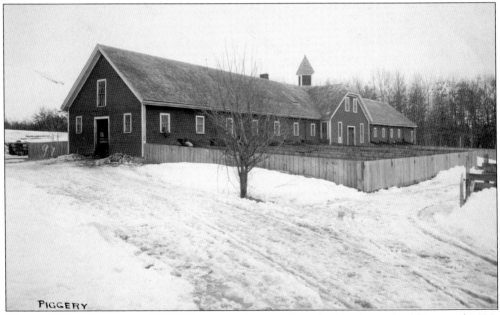

The farm also operated a piggery, which was located near the almshouse building until 1890, when it was moved away from the main structure. In 1910, it was again moved farther east to diminish any detrimental effects on the new tuberculosis hospital built near the pine bank. A study in 1902 revealed about 10 percent of the swine were infected with trichinosis, a parasitic disease, so the infected were slaughtered or quarantined. (Courtesy of Harvard Art Museums/Fogg Museum, Transfer from the Carpenter Center for the Visual Arts, Social Museum Collection.)

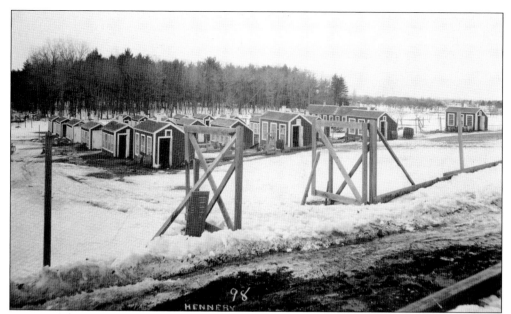

In 1900, the hospital's hens were moved from near the women's asylum to a spot near the piggery. Due to a steady increase in the patient population, the farm animals were likewise increased. In 1916, a new hennery was constructed, and one of the old structures was converted to a brooder, a home for chicks until they are about six weeks old. (Courtesy of Harvard Art Museums/Fogg Museum, Transfer from the Carpenter Center for the Visual Arts, Social Museum Collection.)

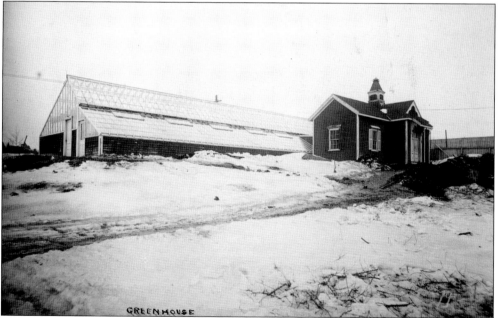

The first greenhouse was in the middle of the main yard until 1894, when it was moved closer to the farm at the southern edge of the campus. By 1899, the greenhouse had cultivated 3,500 plants, and a lean-to was added the following year to increase its capacity. Additional renovations took place in the 1920s and 1930s. (Courtesy of Harvard Art Museums/Fogg Museum, Transfer from the Carpenter Center for the Visual Arts, Social Museum Collection.)

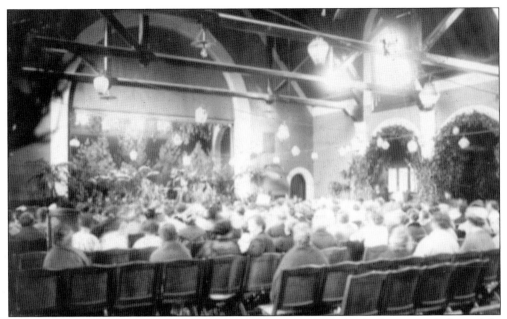

When not working, a patient could spend their time at the chapel, which was regularly used for entertainment and community performances. Due to its active use, an addition was made in 1912, which expanded the seating capacity from 500 to 900 patients. In later years, a two-lane bowling alley was installed in the basement, and the balcony was outfitted with a movie projector. While showing a movie in 1945, the film caught fire, and the bell tower of the Old Chapel was destroyed, never to be rebuilt.

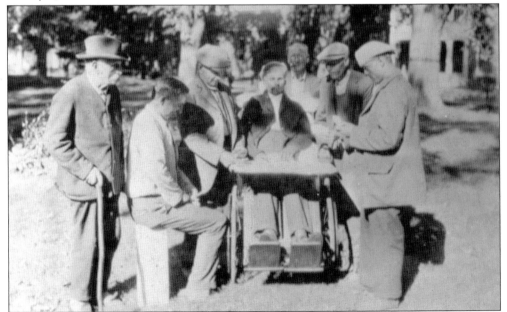

The courtyards served as an escape from overcrowded wards. Patients were instructed in physical fitness exercises in the yards and encouraged to walk the manicured paths. Others gathered with friends to play card games. Any time spent outside was seen as a benefit toward a patient's general happiness at the institution.

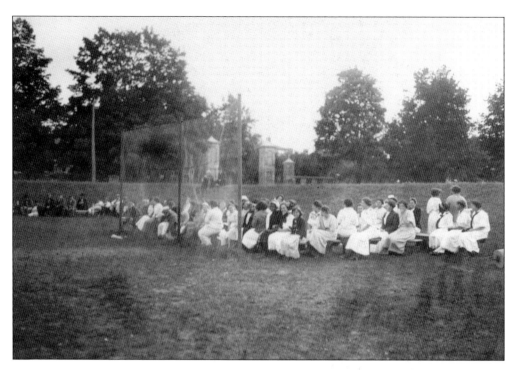

Patients had the opportunity to participate in Fourth of July celebrations, cemetery memorial services, the May Day festival, dances, picnics, and holiday parties. Baseball games were also a popular pastime, with high attendance to cheer on the institutional team. The team was composed of hospital employees who would compete against other state hospitals. The team had its own uniforms, likely made by patients in the laundry department, displaying "S.I." for state infirmary, as seen below in the 1930s.

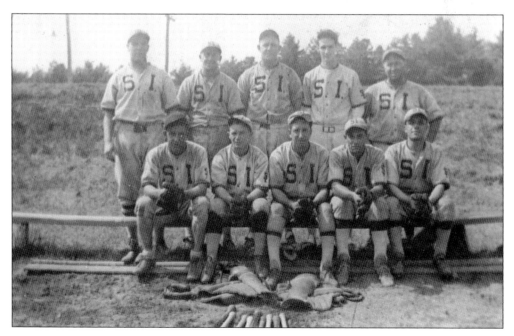

By the beginning of the 20th century, the State Hospital at Tewksbury was providing care for a myriad of patients from chronic cases to convalescents, children to the insane. The initial goal of the institution was to provide care for the neediest of the state who were without permanent residences, but the hospital evolved into much more. Tewksbury developed into a leading research institution, had an immense farm that sustained the campus, and became one of the finest hospitals for tuberculosis, resulting in the bestowment of a gold medal by the International Congress on Tuberculosis in 1908. To reflect its changing priorities, the institution again changed names from the State Hospital at Tewksbury to the State Infirmary at Tewksbury by the Acts of 1909, Chapter 504, Section 98 of the legislature. (Courtesy of Harvard Art Museums/Fogg Museum, Transfer from the Carpenter Center for the Visual Arts, Social Museum Collection.)

Three

CARING FOR THE INFIRM

Communicable diseases can be traced back to the earliest days of human existence, and as the world became more populated and groups interacted, infection spread. Coupled with putrid conditions, diseases like smallpox, tuberculosis, and influenza could annihilate entire communities or result in a worldwide pandemic. Almshouses, mental hospitals, and institutions for the disabled often became breeding grounds for illness and infection. The State Almshouse at Tewksbury was no different, appearing to be a microcosm of whatever disease was ravaging the nation at the time.

Cramped into small, overcrowded wards, sick and well paupers could only be separated so much. Many of the paupers admitted to the almshouse came already in advanced stages of consumption, and diseases became rampant. However, the lead physician and the administration did their best to improve conditions for the infirm. Suitable ventilation throughout wards was a main priority, along with proper heating and ample sunlight, especially for tubercular patients. The medical department deliberately moved away from administering "home remedies" or patent medicines to the sick, instead focusing on bettering the sanitary conditions for overall improvement in the general health of the almshouse.

As the population in the general hospital department expanded, so too did the diseases that became present at Tewksbury State Hospital. Each year, the superintendent or physician would note outbreaks at the institution, with an update on the number infected and any resulting deaths. As more admitted patients required hospital services to address infectious disease or other ailments, the institution's focus shifted from caring for the poor and mentally ill to caring for ailing residents of Massachusetts.

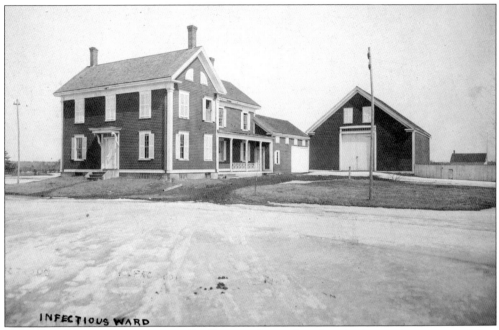

INFECTIOUS WARD

As more sickly paupers and mentally ill were admitted to the almshouse, it was essential to separate the infected from the healthy patients. Several structures served as infectious wards or contagious hospitals in hopes of containing the spread of epidemics that could otherwise devastate the institution and overrun the hospital department. Many of the infectious diseases recorded in annual reports were brought into the institution by newly received patients. Thorough examinations performed at the time of admission would result in a patient being quarantined in one of the infectious wards if they showed signs of disease. (Above, courtesy of Harvard Art Museums/Fogg Museum, Transfer from the Carpenter Center for the Visual Arts, Social Museum Collection.)

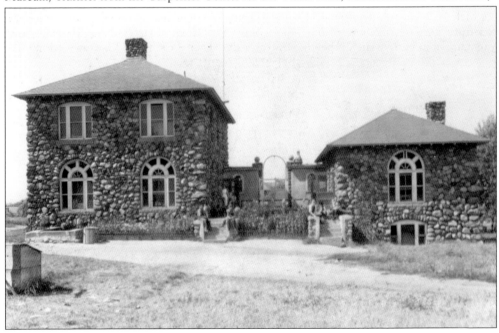

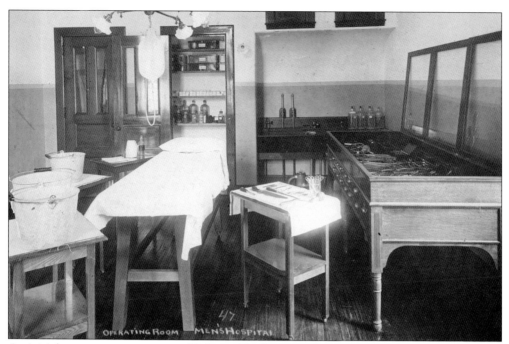

An initial patient examination could also yield a diagnosis that required surgical intervention for improvement and eventual discharge. The earliest surgical procedures began in 1874 and continued to advance over the next two decades until it became its own subset of the medical department. In 1893, around 350 surgical operations were performed on men in the institution, the most common being urethroplasty. Below, Dr. Farrgaes is pictured alongside Elizabeth McCausland and Linda Nase, both graduates of the Training School for Nurses, in the operating room of the Male Hospital. The case holding the surgical instruments is on display at the Public Health Museum. By 1901, hospital administrators acknowledged the shortcomings of the operating rooms within the Male Hospital and the Female Hospital as being too small and ill-equipped, suggesting the construction of one main surgical building. (Above, courtesy of Harvard Art Museums/Fogg Museum, Transfer from the Carpenter Center for the Visual Arts, Social Museum Collection.)

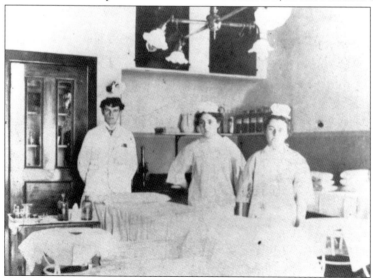

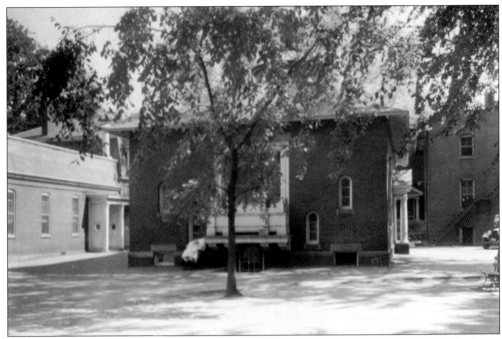

The new surgical building was in the southeast corner of the old quadrangle between the Long Asylum and the Male Hospital. It was constructed of brick with terra-cotta partitions and iron girders, with cement arches to support the floor. The building boasted operating and etherizing rooms, two recovery rooms, sterilizing rooms, a lavatory, and a surgeon's suite. Having an exclusive surgical facility allowed for an increase in the amount of surgical work performed, which surpassed 1,000 operations annually by 1906. This included operations performed on patients in the hospital department, the outpatient department, and the department for the insane.

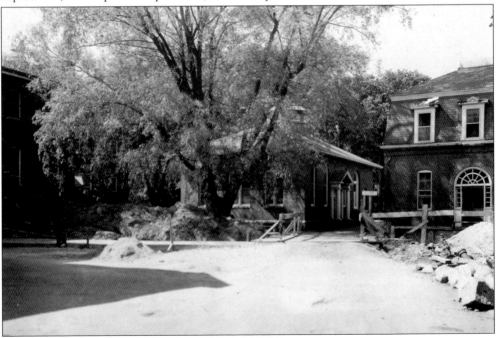

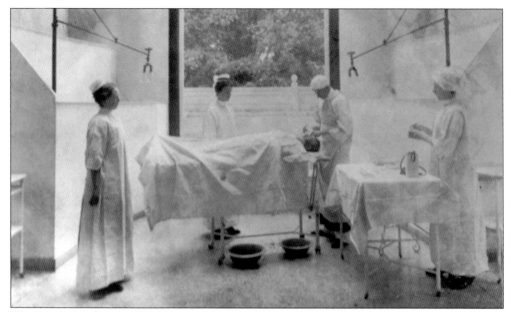

The hospital and surgical functions of the State Hospital continued to grow. In 1914, the general hospital department admitted 7,625 cases. Of that number, 2,404 were reported as surgical, with 614 operations completed within the year. Around 1,000 of the total surgical cases and 85 of the operations were related to eye, ear, nose, and throat conditions. Consequently, the hospital administration hired Dr. Thomas H. Odeneal, a specialist in that field, to attend to patients suffering from these diseases.

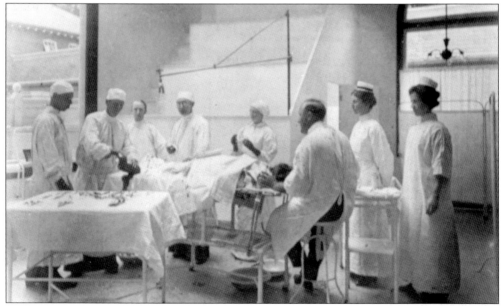

Although much of the surgical procedures performed were meant to remedy a particular disease, the surgical department also handled outpatient cases, which could range from a dog bite to a gunshot wound. Seen here in 1915, Dr. John C. Lindsay is removing a bullet from a patient's foot with the supervision of other doctors and nurses. The operating room was regularly used as an amphitheater to train interns and nurses in surgical care.

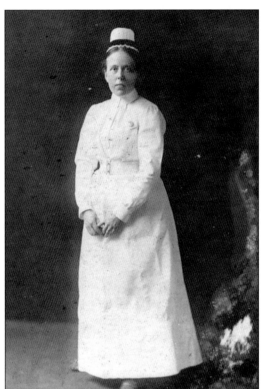

The nurse training school at the State Almshouse at Tewksbury was spearheaded by Clara V. Stevens, who became head nurse in 1891. The training included regular lectures, bedside instruction, and recitation. Nurses gained experience in caring for men, women, and children in a hospital setting, as well as caring for the mentally ill and consumptives.

In 1896, the Training School for Nurses issued its first diplomas to four women, Lillie Fletcher, Albina M. Manning, Heathy Stewart, and Nellie S. Redmond. From there, applications for admission to the nursing program soared, and in 1898, the nursing program was extended from two to three years to provide students with a broader field of experience and usefulness.

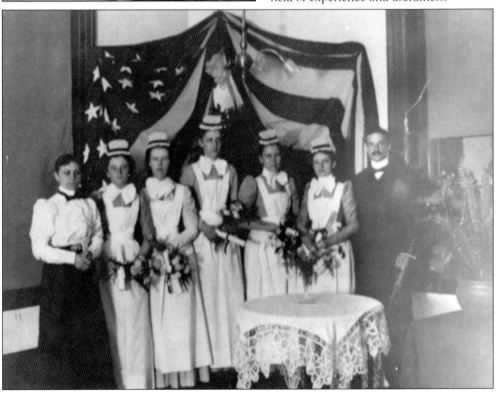

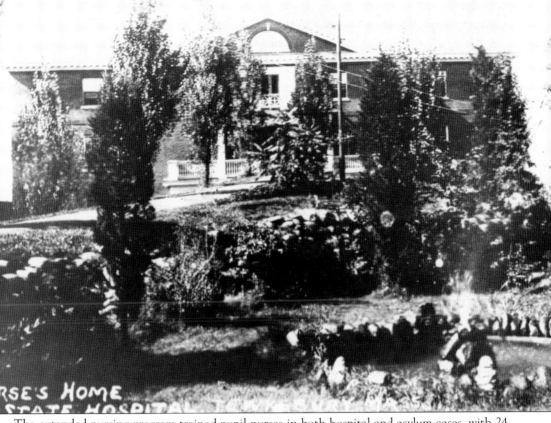

HALL 1
1903

RSE'S HOME
STATE HOSPITAL

The extended nursing program trained pupil nurses in both hospital and asylum cases, with 24 months spent in the hospitals and 12 months in the asylum. Due to the large number of annual hospital admissions, student nurses had exposure to an array of acute and chronic diseases, as well as surgical operations and infectious diseases. The asylum department trained nurses in the various forms and stages of mental disease. With clinical instruction and lectures combined, a graduate would leave as a more efficient nurse, well suited to take positions as heads of departments at Tewksbury or other similar institutions. Student nurses also received compensation for their time in the training school. Nurses in their first six months received $12 per month, $15 per month for the next six months, $17.50 per month for the second year, and $20 per month for the third year. If selected as head of a department, a nurse would make between $25 and $30 per month. They were also provided lodging in the newly constructed Nurses Home.

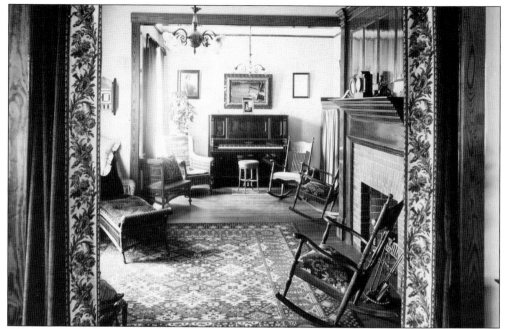

The almshouse administration requested an appropriation in 1896 from the state legislature to construct a home for nurses in order to accommodate students in the training school. The Nurses Home, or Nurses Hall No. 1, cost a total of $20,000 to build and was designed with 40 single rooms for female attendants and nurses to live on-site. It was situated a distance from other buildings to promote physical recuperation after confinement with the sick in the hospital wards and mental recovery from continuous contact with the insane. The Nurses Home was the first to be provided to student nurses among the state institutions. (Above, courtesy of Harvard Art Museums/Fogg Museum, Transfer from the Carpenter Center for the Visual Arts, Social Museum Collection.)

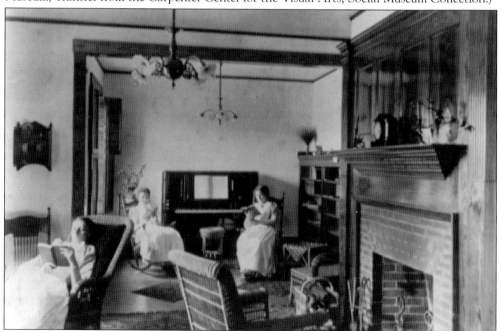

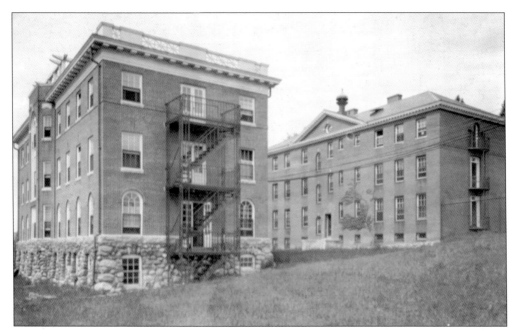

As the training school grew and more nurses and female attendants were added to the staff, it became necessary to provide additional housing for nurses. An appropriation in 1909 allowed for the construction of a second home for nurses just west of the existing Nurses Home, providing an additional 40 private rooms. An annex was later added to connect Nurses Hall No. 1 and Nurses Hall No. 2.

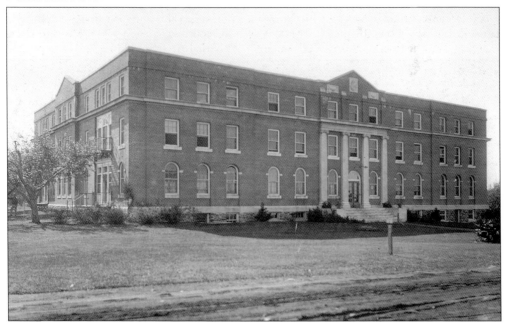

Another home for nurses was requested in 1913, as there was already great overcrowding in the quarters used for nurses, teachers, and matrons, making it almost impossible to add the necessary nursing staff to meet the increasing number of admissions. Nurses Hall No. 3 accommodated an additional 100 nurses for a cost of $70,000.

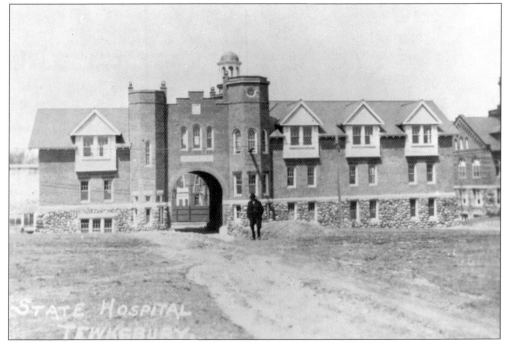

Although female nurses made up the bulk of early employees, men were also employed as physicians, attendants, and officers. A building was erected in 1905 to house 40 male officers. Southgate, as it came to be known, enclosed the southeast corner of the campus. The wooden gates were locked at night, and the only way to enter after hours was with permission of the gatekeeper.

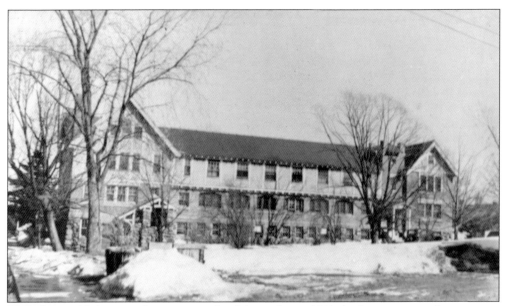

With the establishment of a training school for males in 1911, further accommodations were needed for male employees. Just outside Southgate, another building for male employees was completed in 1914 with a capacity of 40 beds. The officers' quarters were designed by John A. Fox in the Tudor Revival style.

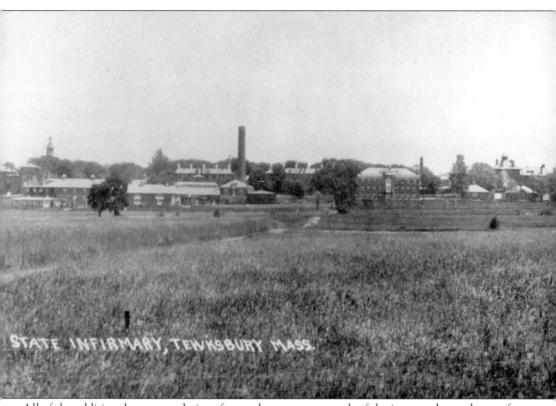

STATE INFIRMARY, TEWKSBURY MASS.

All of the additional accommodations for employees were a result of the increased prevalence of infectious disease at Tewksbury. Each year there were some epidemics present in the almshouse, hospital, or insane departments, ranging from smallpox to scarlet fever, mumps, and a kind of "land scurvy" that spread rapidly and resulted in gangrene or even death. The early 1900s saw a greater focus on caring for patients with contagious diseases, which led to a name change in 1909 from the State Hospital at Tewksbury to the State Infirmary at Tewksbury to differentiate it in comparison to other state institutions.

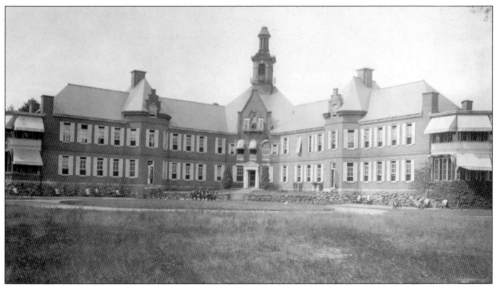

Tuberculosis, or consumption, as it was commonly referred to, emerged in the early 20th century as the dominant concern within the field of public health, and many cases were sent to Tewksbury. The administration responded by constructing a hospital for consumptives in 1899. This hospital, later named the Bancroft Male Tuberculosis Hospital after board of trustees member Cecil F.P. Bancroft, was specifically designed and arranged to provide ample fresh air and sunlight to aid in treatment of consumption. Situated in the pine grove east of the main buildings across Livingston Street, the hospital site was carefully selected based on its sandy soil, sun, and surroundings, and great care went into its construction.

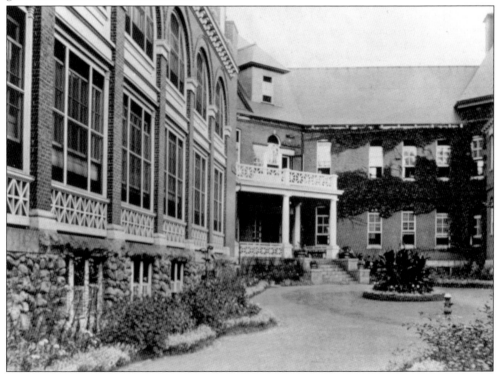

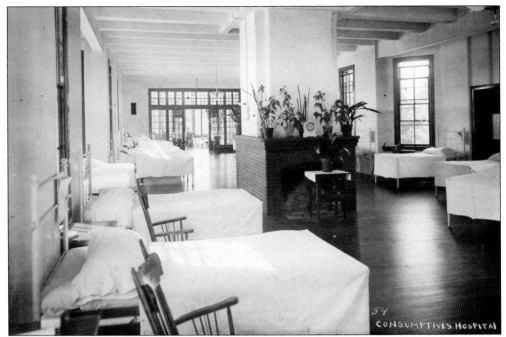

Bancroft was built to accommodate 100 male patients classified in four different wards based on severity of disease. The building was constructed to allow for every bed to be situated near a window for abundant sunlight at all times of the day, and each ward had access to its own large sunroom. Within one year of the consumptive hospital being open, the number of cases of tuberculosis reached 400, with these patients accounting for the largest percentage of institutional deaths. In 1903, there were 489 cases of tuberculosis, and 150 perished. (Both, courtesy of Harvard Art Museums/Fogg Museum, Transfer from the Carpenter Center for the Visual Arts, Social Museum Collection.)

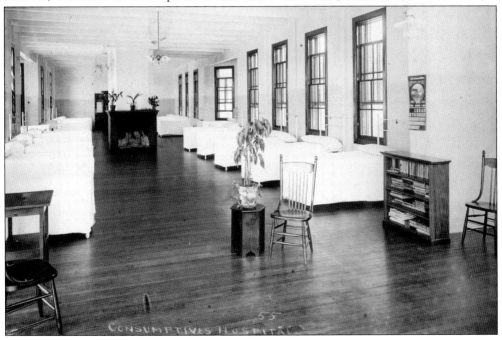

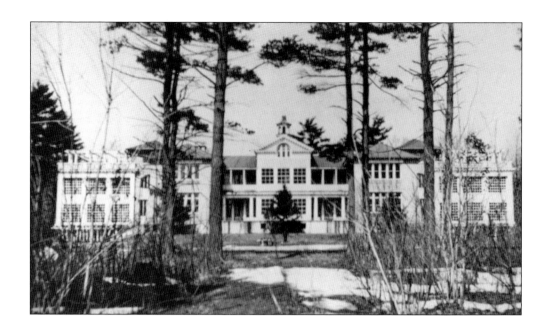

As tuberculosis became more prevalent and fatal in Massachusetts, Tewksbury administration requested an appropriation for the construction of a female consumptive hospital for $25,000. This hospital, later named the Fiske House after board of trustees member Sarah D. Fiske, was erected in 1906 on the hill to the south of the water reservoir surrounded by young white pine and oak trees. By the end of its opening day on January 1, 1908, the Fiske House had already reached its capacity of 40 patients. By 1909, the board of trustees already indicated a need for expansion.

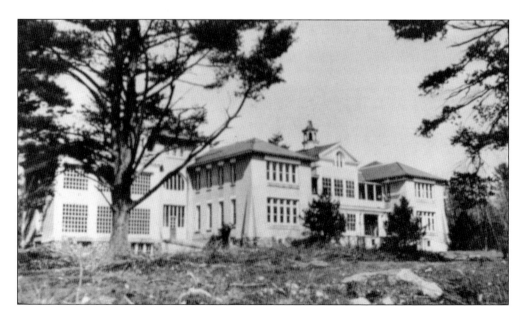

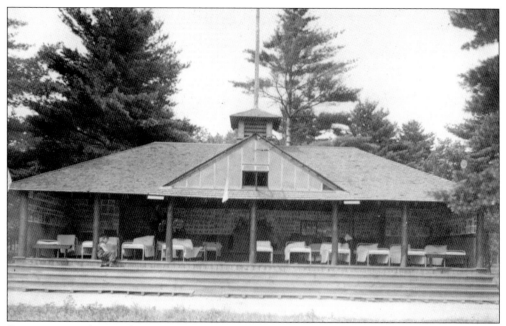

Some overcrowding in the consumptive hospitals was remedied by the addition of plain open-air camps near Bancroft. The first was added in 1904, with two more camps erected in 1905 and 1906. Each housed 20 patients, who would elect to inhabit these quarters. One such camp was later utilized by boys who were part of the children's ward.

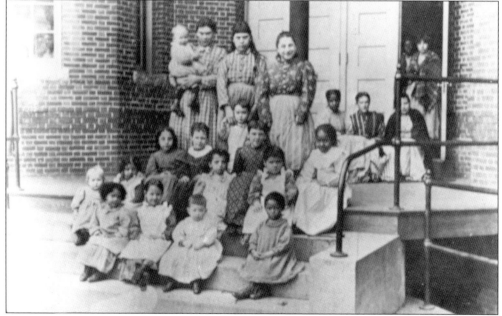

Children were no strangers to the institution at Tewksbury. Primarily sent to the State Almshouse at Monson to receive an education, some children remained in Tewksbury if their mother was a patient, if they were afflicted with an illness, or if they were diagnosed as feeble-minded. The children were confined to a ward within the Women's Dormitory before a more suitable structure was erected.

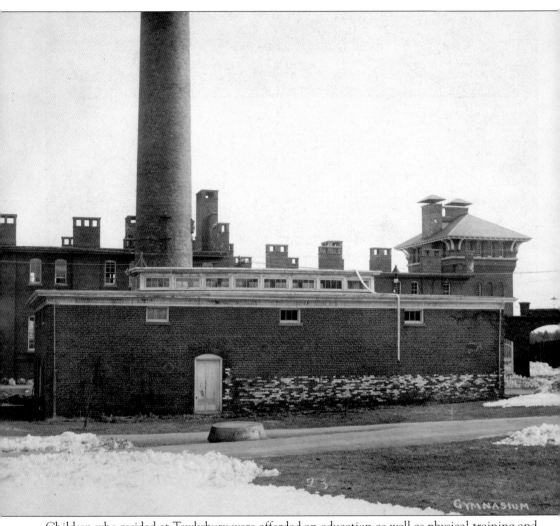

Children who resided at Tewksbury were afforded an education as well as physical training and recreational activities. Girls spent their days in class and their evenings between sewing lessons, gymnastics, or dance classes. Boys alternated days between school work and the manual training shop, and their evenings were spent receiving either military training or athletic work. Efforts were made to provide an engaging and beneficial space for the children in hopes of them "finding themselves and acquiring their bearings in regard to responsibility," according to the Annual Report of 1919. (Courtesy of Harvard Art Museums/Fogg Museum, Transfer from the Carpenter Center for the Visual Arts, Social Museum Collection.)

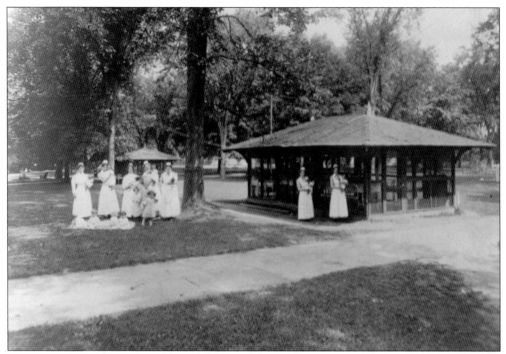

The children at the State Hospital were also affected by the various epidemics in any given year. Scarlet fever, measles, and whooping-cough all contributed to a large death toll among children in the early years of the institution. But measures were put into place to try to provide for the children's health. Much like the insane wards and tubercular patients, summerhouses and outdoor recreation provided opportunities for sunlight and fresh air to infants and young children.

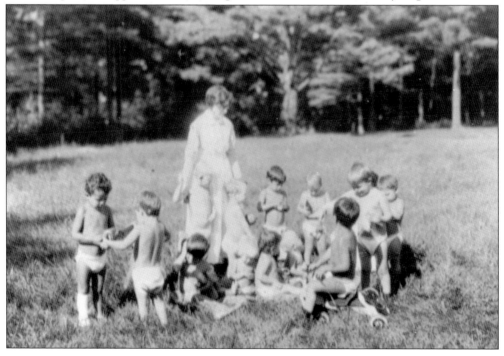

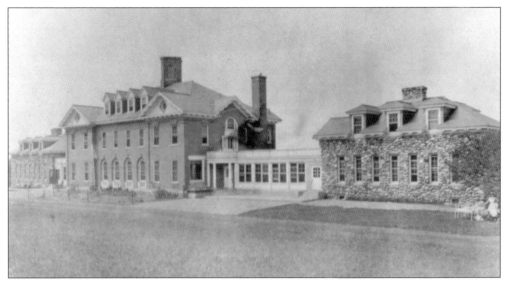

To reduce overcrowding in the Women's Dormitory and to provide more individualized care, Superintendent Nichols recommended the construction of a children's building outside the confines of the main campus. In 1907, the legislature approved $30,000 for the construction of the Children's Hospital designed to accommodate 100 beds.

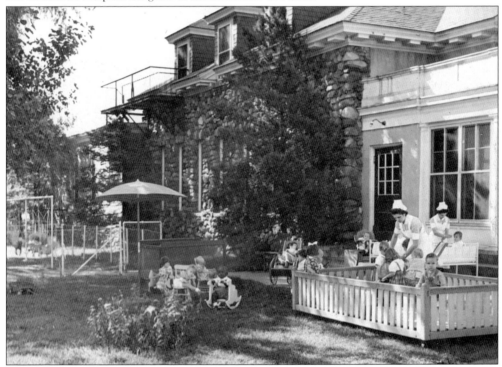

Occupied in May 1910, the Children's Hospital quickly exceeded its capacity. The Annual Report of 1911 noted the "increasing number of children and minors during the last year, until the number has reached 400 under the age of 21 years, and among this increase especially, have been a large proportion of feeble-minded cases." Many children were placed back into the Women's Dormitory or housed in temporary open-air camps.

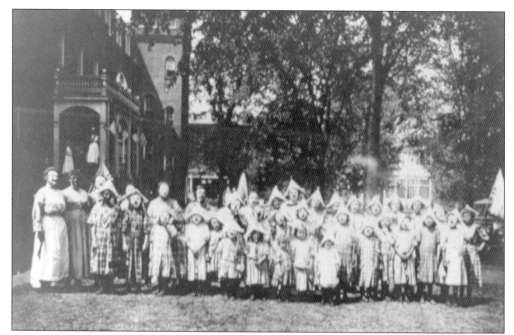

Although institutionalized children experienced many hardships, the staff tried to provide opportunities for enjoyment when possible. The children dressed in comic and grotesque costumes to participate in the "parade of horribles" on the Fourth of July, a 19th-century tradition started in Massachusetts and celebrated in parts of New England.

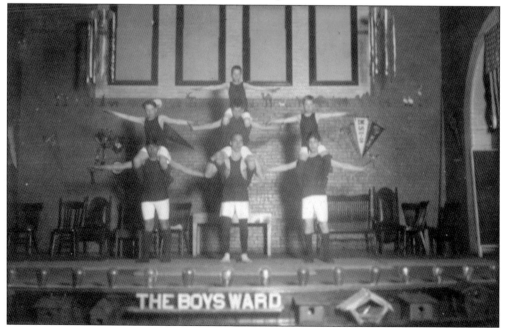

Children received instruction in physical education through dancing classes, drills, and exercises for both boys and girls, and participation in other outdoor pastimes. They also performed plays, vaudevilles, and musical concerts for patients. The boys' ward exhibited acts of physical fitness and gymnastics as entertainment in 1917.

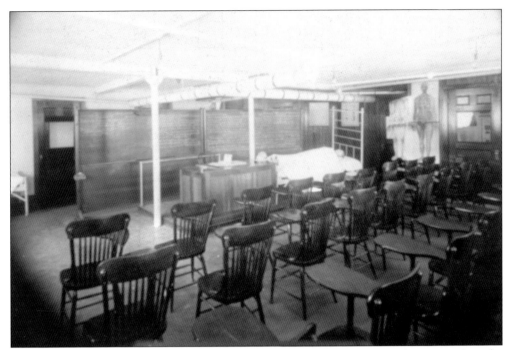

Although extracurricular activities were plentiful, they were but a temporary distraction from the swelling number of patients being admitted with infectious diseases. As early as 1904, students in the Training School for Nurses were required to take courses in bacteriology and pathology to better understand the cause and effects of the diseases afflicting their patients.

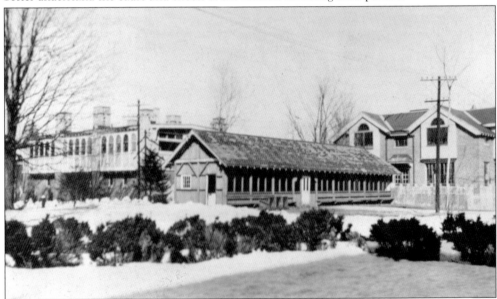

Due to advances in medical science and the thousands of hospital cases requiring pathological investigation, Superintendent Nichols urged the legislature in 1912 to fund a clinical laboratory. Completed in 1914, the lab (left) was equipped with space for postmortem examinations, consulting rooms, a large laboratory for general pathology, and two smaller sections for biological chemistry and bacteriology, as well as office space for staff.

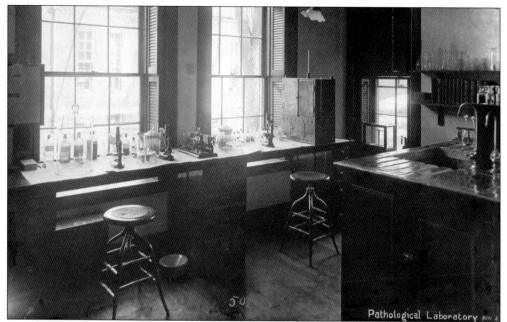

The laboratory department came to be of paramount importance as the State Infirmary at Tewksbury shifted to a public health institution. In addition to autopsies and examinations of blood, urine, or bodily fluids for diagnostic purposes, the laboratory broadened its scope to focus on the study of conditions in hopes of suggesting possible new treatment plans for patients. Early tests for pregnancy were carried out in the lab, as well as experiments into acute nephritis, rabies, and tuberculosis. Other tests administered to patients included the Wassermann test for syphilis, the Schwartz test for gonorrhea, and a new test to diagnose infantile paralysis that was developed at Tewksbury. (Both, courtesy of Harvard Art Museums/Fogg Museum, Transfer from the Carpenter Center for the Visual Arts, Social Museum Collection.)

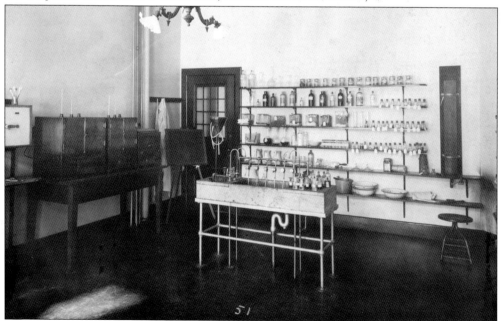

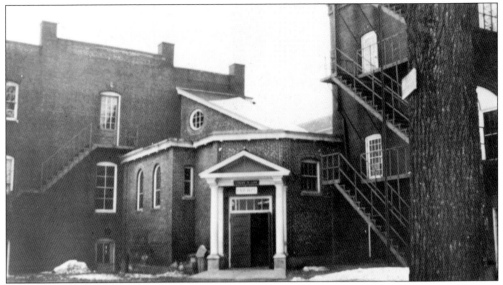

An X-ray apparatus was purchased for the hospital department in 1899 to further aid in accurate diagnoses by physicians. By 1915, Tewksbury had two x-ray machines on-site, and a new one was purchased in 1918 for $1,916.65. Its frequent use warranted a formalized X-ray department, which was led by Dr. Frederick E. Twitchell beginning in 1918. Dr. Twitchell was also the head of the dental department.

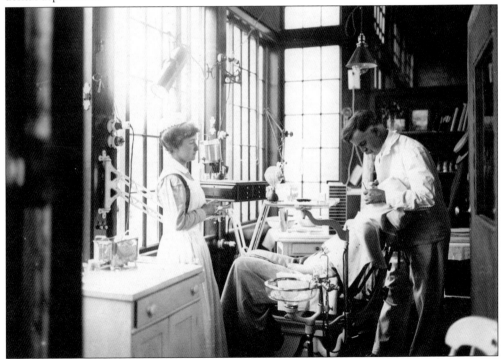

Dr. Frederick E. Twitchell was officially appointed to the medical staff in 1912 to lead the dental department. In his first year, Dr. Twitchell performed dental work on 500 patients across the entire inmate population, including cleaning and polishing of teeth, fillings, root canals, and extractions. For many patients, it was likely the first time they received a dental examination.

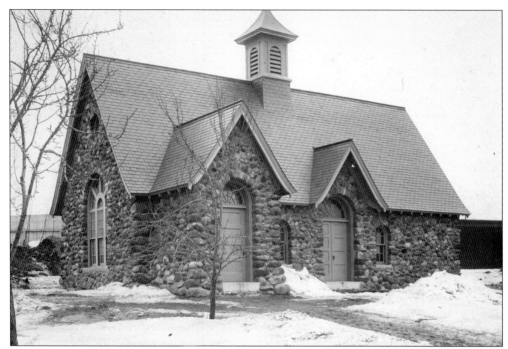

Even with the medical advances brought to the State Infirmary at Tewksbury in the early 20th century, many patients succumbed to their ailments. Accordingly, the hospital administration saw the need to erect a mortuary chapel on the grounds. The structure had two distinct uses, to hold funeral services and to act as a morgue. During construction, pipes were laid from the main cold storage system to the mortuary chapel in order to provide refrigeration. Built entirely of fieldstone, the chapel was completed in January 1903. (Courtesy of Harvard Art Museums/Fogg Museum, Transfer from the Carpenter Center for the Visual Arts, Social Museum Collection.)

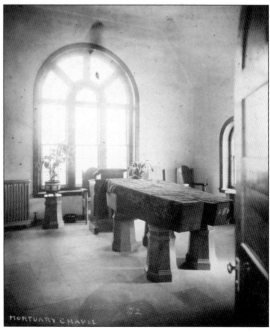

It was thought that the mortuary chapel would be effective in adding comfort to the last visit of friends of deceased patients. The chapel was placed near the Southgate, which was typically used by employees, not patients. This would limit the frequency of patients seeing bodies of the deceased transported to the Pines Cemetery across Livingston Street. (Courtesy of Harvard Art Museums/Fogg Museum, Transfer from the Carpenter Center for the Visual Arts, Social Museum Collection.)

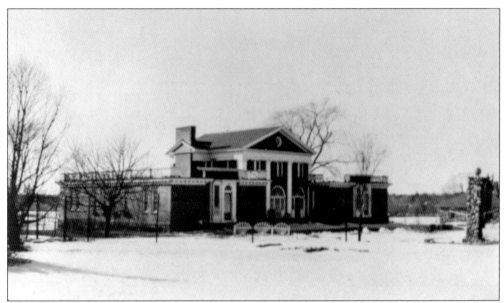

Although a relatively self-sustaining community, the State Infirmary at Tewksbury was not immune to the problems affecting the nation. As the United States entered World War I, admissions were high and nursing staff and physicians were low due to the draft. This ushered in the establishment of the School of Practical Nursing in 1920 to produce "relief nurses" for the infirmary. The School for Practical Nursing replaced the three-year Training School for Nurses, which graduated its last class in 1942. In total, the Training School for Nurses graduated nearly 700 nurses over 50 years. The succeeding School for Practical Nursing operated its training and home care center out of the Women's Special Ward, completed in 1913.

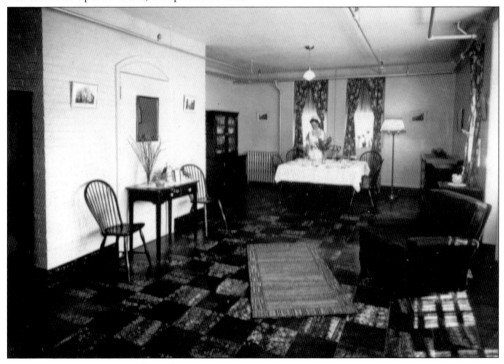

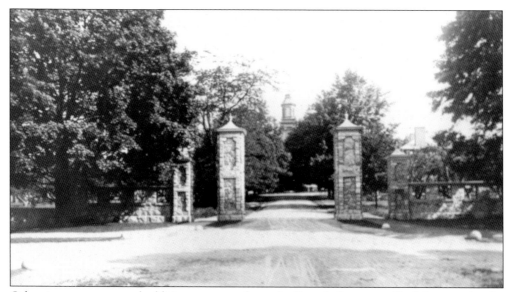

Other improvements and additions were made to the State Infirmary at Tewksbury under the leadership of Superintendent Nichols. One was the construction of a new main entrance on East Street in 1913. The entrance consisted of four large stone pillars that connected to a stone wall that encompassed the campus's main structures.

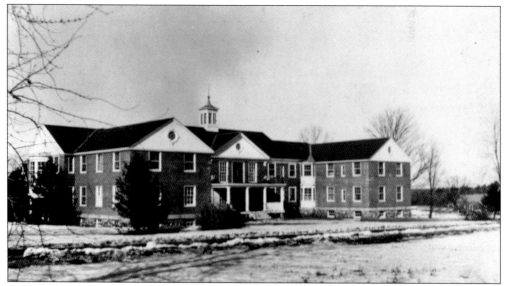

Unlike the new entrance, other additions were out of necessity, not novelty. The administration began requesting a building to house married couples in the early 1920s. In 1931, an appropriation was finally made to construct new employee quarters for $74,000. The building was designed with 24 two-bed suites of rooms with reception halls on each of the two floors.

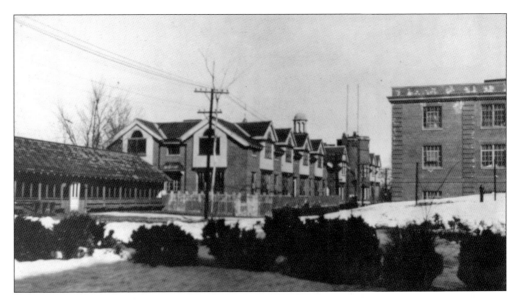

Prior to 1932, industrial work was performed in various buildings across the campus. The introduction of an industrial building allowed for industrial activities to take place under one roof. Opened on June 1, 1932, the building boasted three well-lit floors accommodating machinery work on the first floor, textile work on the second floor, and occupational therapy on the third floor. Ground was broken for the brick storehouse in 1934, a project commissioned by the Public Works Administration and erected by D.W. Walker of Lowell for $149,000. The new structure filled a dire need of the infirmary by bringing all groceries, clothing, and hospital supplies into one location. (Below, courtesy of Harvard Art Museums/Fogg Museum, Transfer from the Carpenter Center for the Visual Arts, Social Museum Collection.)

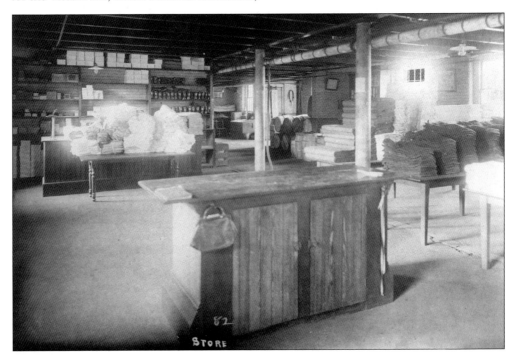

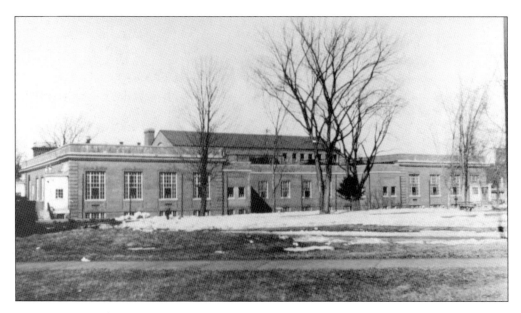

Due to excessive demands on the kitchens, dining rooms, and dietary services, and the sheer age of the domestic building, a new structure was essential to serve the growing patient population. In 1934, the construction of a new dietary building was approved by the Public Works Administration and brought almost all dining rooms and kitchens under one roof. Contracted for $520,000, the new cafeteria could seat 1,101 and was equipped with a mammoth kitchen, a pasteurizing and milk bottling room, a fish department, storage rooms and refrigerators, and a most impressive bakery.

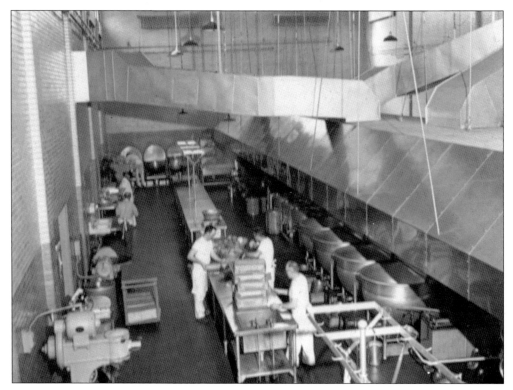

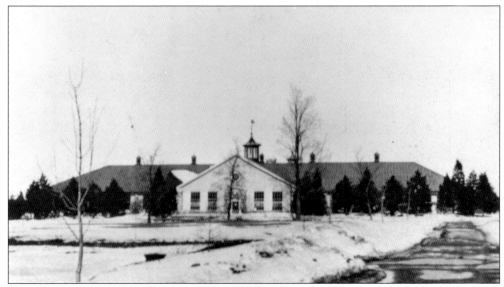

To alleviate the constant overcrowding within the men's pavilion, a new building for men was completed in 1929 on the edge of a hill at the southeast part of the campus. Made of fieldstone, hollow tile, and cement, Stonecroft was designed in three sections, two of which served as dormitories connected by one large intersecting living room.

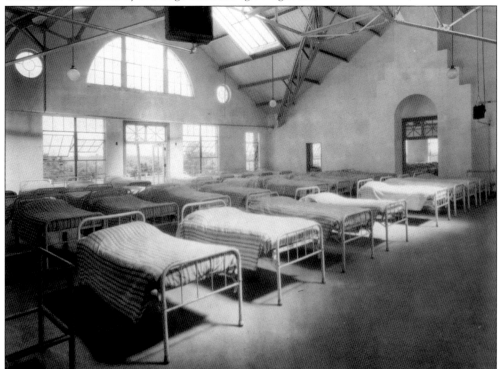

Stonecroft could hold up to 384 men, and the young or more physically fit patients were selected to live there to separate them from the more aged or feeble patients in the general hospital department. The building was outfitted with bunk beds and rows of large windows to provide fresh air to patients, especially those with tuberculosis.

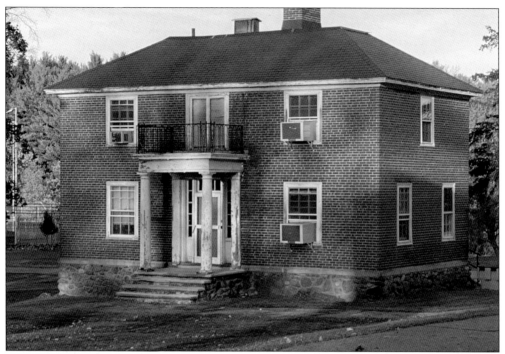

Originally requested in 1922, a home for the assistant superintendent was constructed shortly thereafter for about $19,000. Built in the Colonial Revival style, the house was directly across from the Superintendent's Home and served as residence to the assistant superintendent and his family. Later, the building was named the Milot House in honor of Charles Milot, the chief engineer of the hospital for many years. (Ashlynn Rickord Werner.)

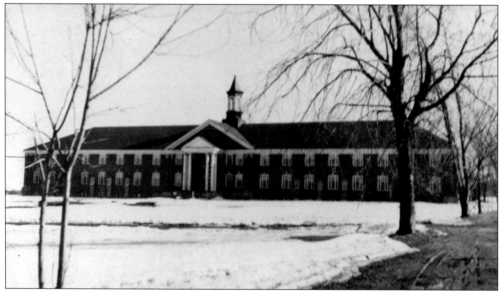

Adjacent to Stonecroft, a new hospital to accommodate 400 patients was constructed in 1939 on the former site of the boys' camp. The Dr. John Holyoke Nichols Infirmary, or the Nichols Building, was named in honor of Dr. Nichols, who served as superintendent of the institution for 38 years.

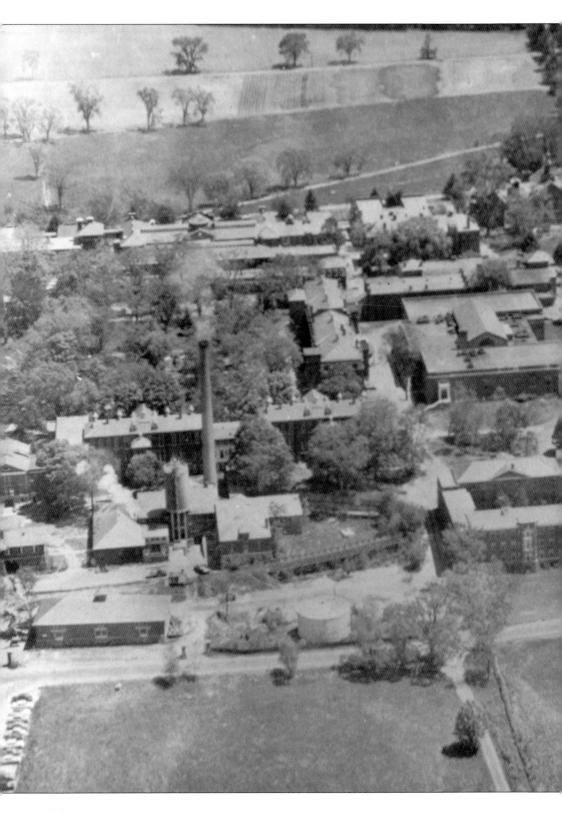

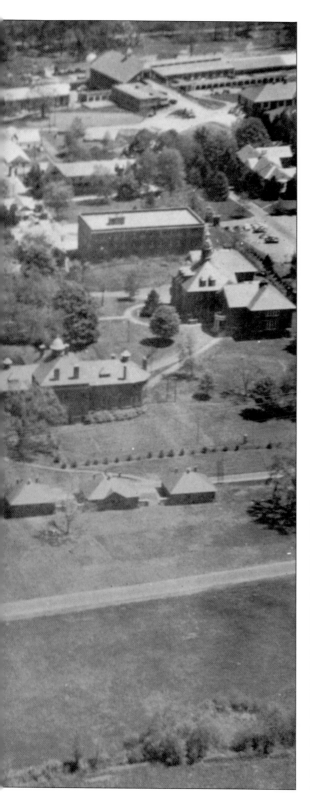

In 1939, the institution again changed names to best reflect its predominant functions. Henceforth known as the Tewksbury State Hospital and Infirmary, it was acknowledged as the eighth largest institution of all classifications and the second largest general hospital in the United States by the American Hospital Association in 1939. The campus had reached its pinnacle by 1940, with over 50 buildings designed to care for its diverse patient population as well as its staff and administrators. Tewksbury State Hospital and Infirmary continued to serve the mentally ill, alcoholics, acute and chronic hospital cases, and patients with contagious diseases under the Department of Public Welfare until 1959.

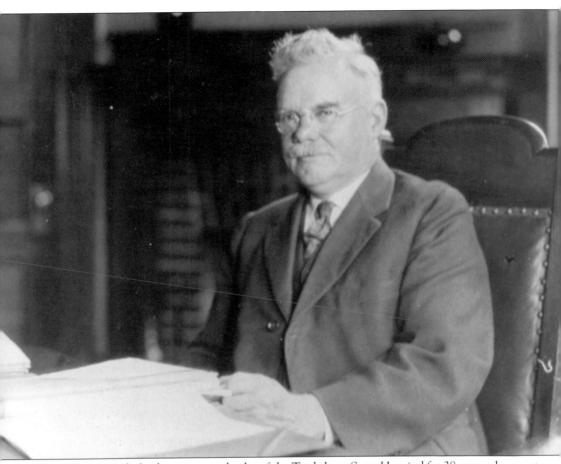

Dr. John H. Nichols, the enigmatic leader of the Tewksbury State Hospital for 38 years who spent a total of 44 years serving the institution, was the catalyst for positive change and expansion of the campus to best serve those in need. Most of his goals had been accomplished in whole or in part by the time of his retirement: hospitals were built for convalescents and tubercular patients; updates were made to wooden structures; first-class fireproofing was installed to standards of the time; housing was built for nurses, attendants, physicians, and administrators to provide for their safety, health, and happiness; impressive advances in medical research and treatment were made; and equity and justice for the best interests of the state, the citizen, and the patient were ensured. His remarkable tenure as superintendent positioned the institution for a bright future.

Four

CARING FOR THE AFFLICTED

As the United States grappled with the Great Depression, emphasis was placed on supplying unemployment benefits and "old age" assistance to those affected by the economic downturn. The Social Security Act was introduced, and access to adequate medical care became a contentious issue. By the 1960s, funding from the federal government helped support states in providing medical assistance to residents who otherwise could not afford it. Medication to treat infections and mental illness became commonplace, while compulsory vaccinations led to the near eradication of many diseases that patients were treated for at the State Infirmary at Tewksbury.

With a shift to the Department of Public Health in 1959, operations at Tewksbury Hospital experienced some major changes. No longer were psychiatric patients admitted, along with those infected with smallpox or other diseases dangerous to public health such as tuberculosis. The services that would continue to be offered included treatment of patients with cardiovascular, pulmonary, renal, neurological, diabetic, and arthritic diseases. The Tewksbury Hospital also offered surgical operations, obstetric and pediatric departments, an active laboratory, and specialty clinics for eye, ear, nose, and throat diseases.

As one of the oldest continuously operational state institutions in Massachusetts, the Tewksbury Hospital continues to care for the most vulnerable in the state. While the hospital itself offers numerous clinical and specialty services, the historic campus is also home to a number of government agencies, clinical programs, and the Public Health Museum.

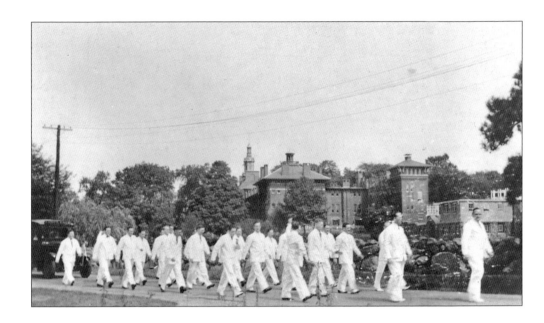

An impressive campus encompassing around 900 acres, the State Infirmary at Tewksbury was synonymous with the town of Tewksbury. Many local residents who did not live on campus were involved with the institution, from donating to the library to providing entertainment for patients. When the town of Tewksbury celebrated its 200th anniversary on August 25–27, 1934, the State Infirmary participated in the town exhibition and flower show and formed the second division of the parade with representation from the board of trustees, the medical staff, clerical force, nurses in uniform, and all of the departments of the infirmary, which included around 300 employees. Patients were also able to enjoy the festivities as much as possible with use of the athletic field and grounds as part of the celebration.

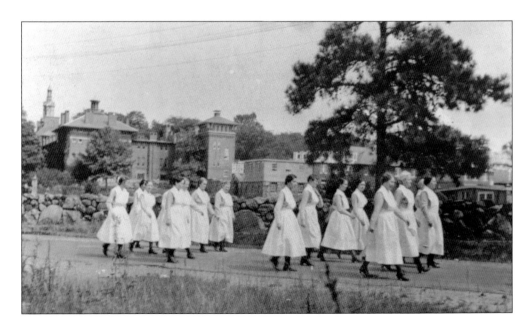

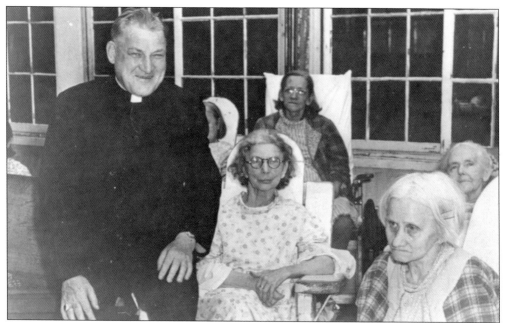

The religious life of the institution was also vibrant, for those who participated. Religious instruction was provided for those of the Catholic, Jewish, and Protestant faiths, and Italian residents were attended by the Franciscan fathers. Notable religious figures like Richard Cardinal Cushing, archbishop of Boston, made periodic visits to the Tewksbury State Hospital and Infirmary to visit with patients and staff.

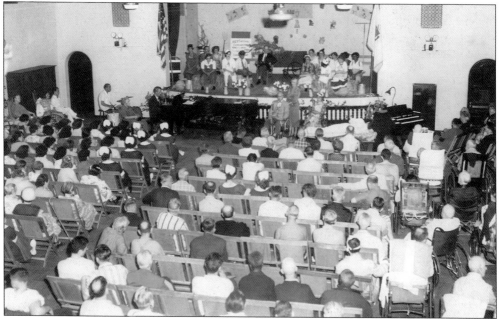

Although the patient population was aging, especially in the mental ward, recreational opportunities continued to be provided in the Old Chapel and athletic fields. More movies were shown, and bingo nights became popular. Other offerings included holiday parties and sleigh rides at Christmas and plays and musical performances put on by members of the community.

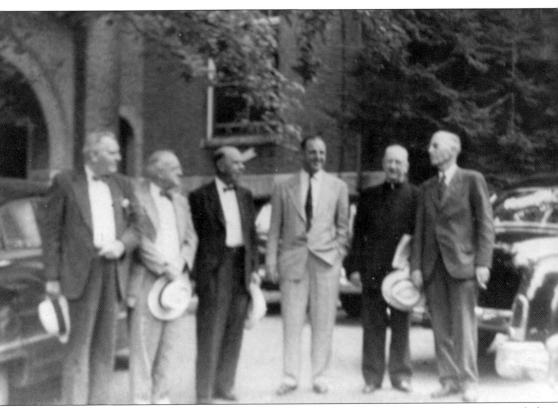

By the second half of the 20th century, state institutions were predominantly serving custodial cases. Revisions to old age assistance and disability assistance laws through the Social Security Act resulted in a shift in the patient population of Tewksbury State Hospital. These changes also affected operations of the board of public welfare, which had been "entangled in a maze of settlement laws, varying reimbursement formulas, and meaningless eligibility restrictions," according to the Sixth Report on Laws of the Commonwealth Relating to Public Welfare by Special Commission to Study and Revise the Laws Relating to Public Welfare, complicating the process of providing public assistance for those requiring state support. By June 30, 1952, the population had dropped to 1,568 patients at Tewksbury in comparison to 2,490 at the highest daily census in 1942 and 3,252 in 1932. Where appropriate, custodial cases were transferred to rest homes or released to their families to provide care.

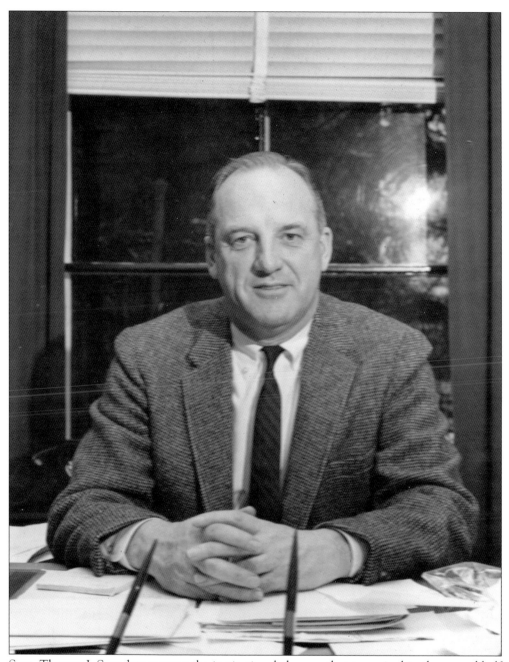

Supt. Thomas J. Saunders oversaw the institutional changes that transpired in the second half of the 20th century. The first superintendent to not have a medical background since Thomas J. Marsh in 1883, Saunders earned his degree in business administration from Holy Cross College. At the onset of World War II, he enlisted in the Navy and served for four years before retiring at the rank of lieutenant commander in 1946. On February 20, 1951, he began his employment with the Tewksbury State Hospital and Infirmary and led the institution for 35 years. Before retiring in 1986, Saunders was named the Tewksbury Chamber of Commerce's Man of the Year, among other awards and recognitions for his dedicated service.

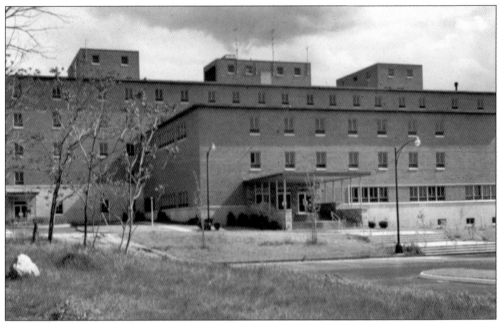

Among the accomplishments during Saunders's time as superintendent was the construction of a new main hospital for the campus in the 1960s, with additions to expand its occupancy in the 1970s. The new facility provided modern convenience for patients and staff and brought many auxiliary functions under one roof. The new medical building was also one of the first structures built under the institution's new name. Enacted in 1959 by the Massachusetts legislature, the Tewksbury State Hospital and Infirmary became simply the Tewksbury Hospital. By the same legislation, the hospital came under the purview of the Department of Public Health, no longer overseen by the Department of Public Welfare, although Tewksbury Hospital still accepted public welfare patients.

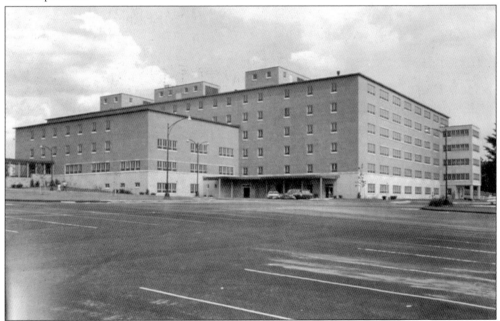

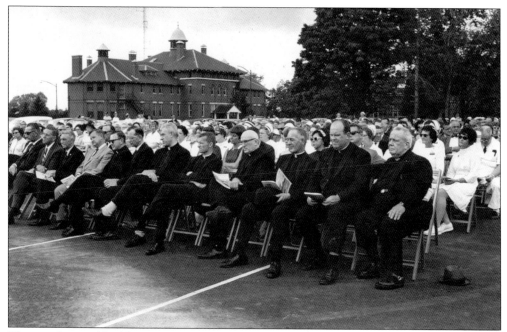

The new hospital building was one of the crowning achievements of Thomas J. Saunders, and members of the medical community recognized that. Therefore, the hospital was designated the Thomas J. Saunders Building in 1976 to honor the superintendent who was responsible for turning the institution into a modern chronic and long-term care facility.

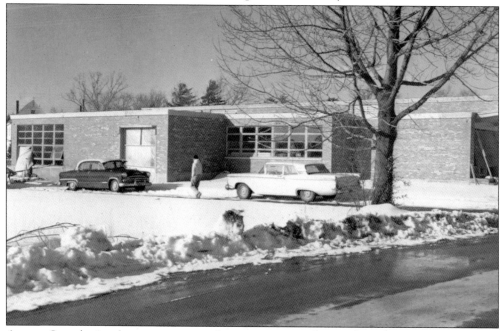

Among Saunders's other successes was the construction of a new laundry facility in the early 1960s to house new washing machines, specifically selected for their labor-saving claims as the patient population involved in domestic work dwindled. Currently, the building is used as the State Office for Pharmacy Services.

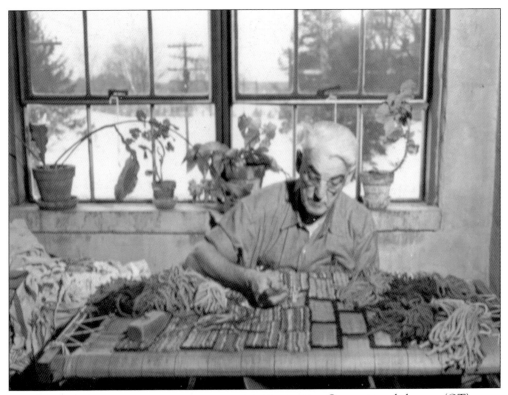

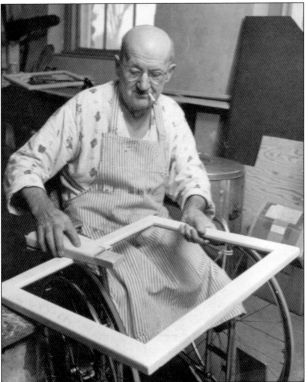

Occupational therapy (OT) at Tewksbury came a long way from the early years of the institution. In the 20th century, the OT department assisted patients in developing, regaining, or improving skills in varying activities. These services took the form of weaving, hooking, rug making, painting, woodworking, furniture repairing and refinishing, model construction, radio repairing, chair caning, knitting, crocheting, and needlework, as noted in the Annual Report of 1953. Over 100 patients benefited from the services of the OT department, and even more enjoyed the holiday parties and dances hosted by OT staff members throughout the year.

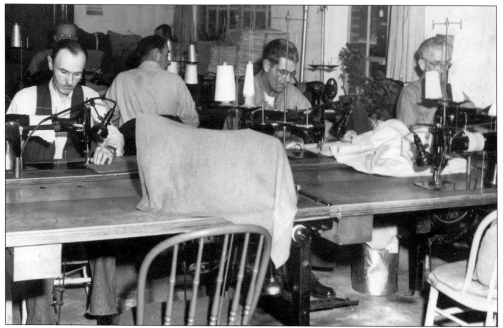

Like occupational therapy, the industrial department was valuable to patients' treatment, but it also was advantageous to Tewksbury Hospital for producing goods to be used by the institution. Saunders recorded that the industrial department manufactured over 40,000 articles of clothing, bedding, or other linens in 1952. Patients who participated in the industrial department also assisted with repairing and hemming clothing, printing cards and programs, and binding books. Skills of printing and book binding were especially useful to the library department, which boasted thousands of books, newspapers, and magazines, many of which were donated by local organizations or community members.

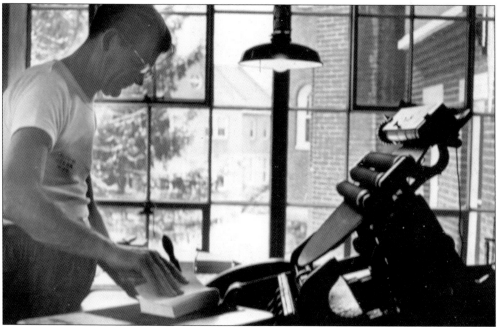

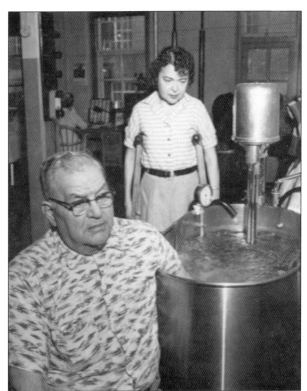

As physical therapy, or physiotherapy as referred to in Annual Reports from the 1950s, became commonplace in hospitals, the Tewksbury Hospital enlisted licensed physiotherapists to address physical functioning for both acute and chronic care patients. A new physical therapy room was situated near the X-ray room in the Saunders Building to embrace an integrative approach to treatment.

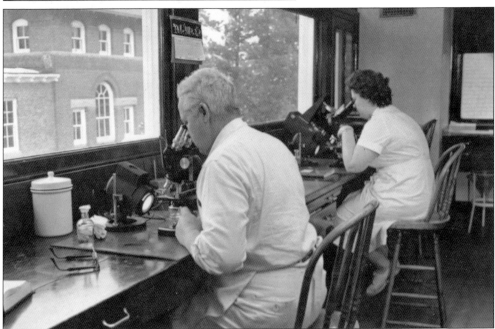

Laboratory services continued to expand after the opening of the lab building in 1914. By the 1950s, the pathological laboratory had several subsections of testing including chemical, serology, hematology, bacteriology, and pathology. Most lab services had transitioned to the Saunders Building by 1970.

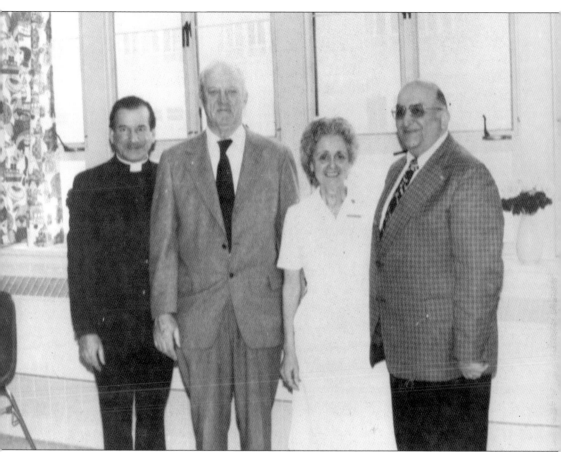

Institutional improvements were not all Thomas J. Saunders was known for during his tenure as superintendent. Saunders did much to positively affect the Tewksbury community. With patient numbers shrinking and a majority of hospital services based out of the Saunders Building, a 900-acre campus seemed excessive, and Saunders was instrumental in convincing the state to return some land to the town. Around 100 acres were eventually ceded back to Tewksbury and became schools, an elderly housing complex, parks, and a senior center.

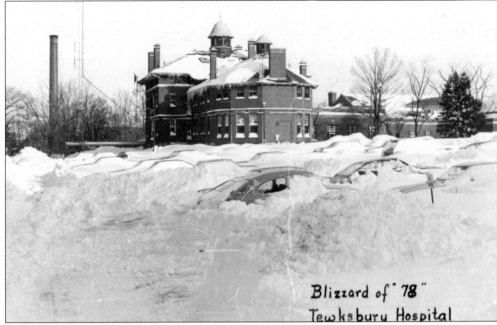

Blizzard of "78"
Tewksbury Hospital

The blizzard of 1978 rocked the Northeastern United States in early February, and Tewksbury Hospital was no exception. The storm dumped a record 27 inches of snow in Boston, burying cars and stranding employees at the hospital. Luckily, staff and nursing students who did not live on-site could pay a nominal fee to stay in a hospital dormitory during inclement weather like the blizzard. This was beneficial to hospital administration, as staff would be able to assist with the cleanup. The snow removal effort was tremendous, as even the farm's payloader struggled with the vast quantity of snow. Eventually, outside help was called in to clear the several dozen vehicles that were trapped.

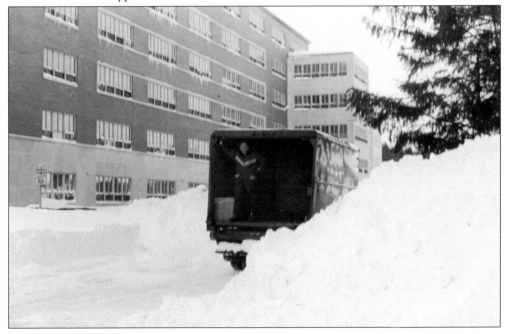

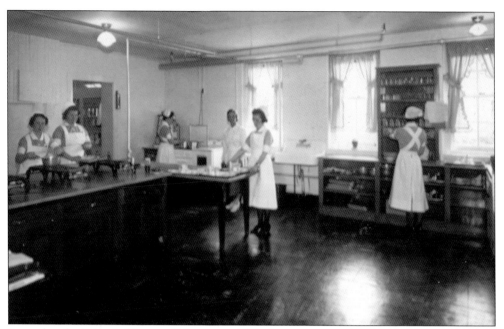

Started as the School of Practical Nursing in 1920, the program produced on average three dozen licensed practical nurses each year well into the 1990s. A benefit to student nurses was that it took only 11 months to complete the program, with ample on-the-job training at the bedsides of patients, unlike similar programs at colleges. The school had many affiliations with other medical and state institutions in Massachusetts, including the Cape Cod Hospital, Gardner State Hospital, Pondville Hospital, Westborough State Hospital, and Westfield State Sanatorium. It was a well-regarded program for fundamental training in nursing, but a $2 million budget cut in 1995 resulted in the School of Practical Nursing getting axed shortly thereafter. The closure saved the Tewksbury Hospital around $400,000.

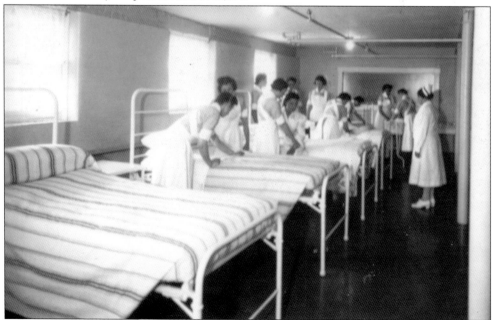

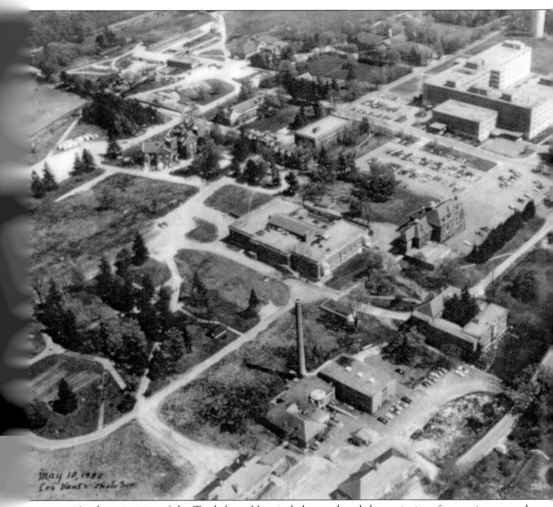

may 10, 1980
Les Vant x Photo Ser

As the priorities of the Tewksbury Hospital changed and the majority of operations were house in the Saunders Building, the dilapidated condition of excess buildings necessitated their razir Among those slated for demolition was the Long Asylum, a pre–Civil War structure that was or of the oldest of those that would be torn down. By the mid-1970s when demolition was comple virtually all of the buildings related to the institution's history as an almshouse were gone. Lucki the structures erected during the major building campaign of the late 1800s and later remaine relatively untouched, maintaining some of the historic character of the campus. Among th remaining buildings, almost all found new tenants. The maintenance buildings on the weste edge continued to serve the remnants of the once expansive institution.

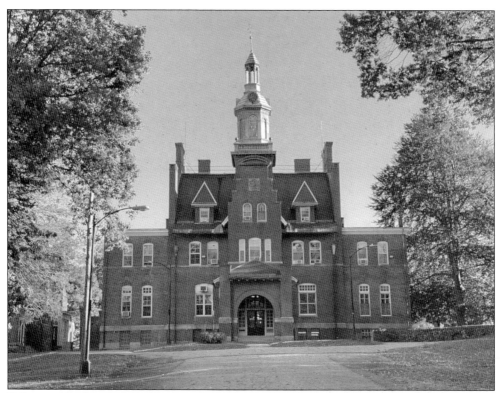

Following the demolition of the original almshouse-era buildings in the 1970s, the campus retained most of its historic structures from the late 1800s. Most notable among them is the striking Old Administration Building, which serves as a focal point of the campus from East Street. The Old Administration Building currently serves as the Northeast Area Office for the Department of Mental Health as well as the home of the Public Health Museum. Upon entering the central entry pavilion, historic "Office Entrance" and "Patients Admitted Downstairs" signs are still visible. Through the main wooden doors are granite steps etched with the names of Dr. Herbert Burr Howard and Dr. John Holyoke Nichols in honor of the two superintendents responsible for the transition of the institution from an almshouse to a hospital. (Above, Ashlynn Rickord Werner.)

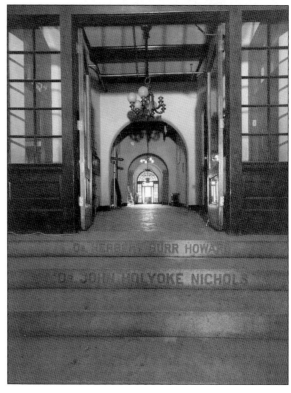

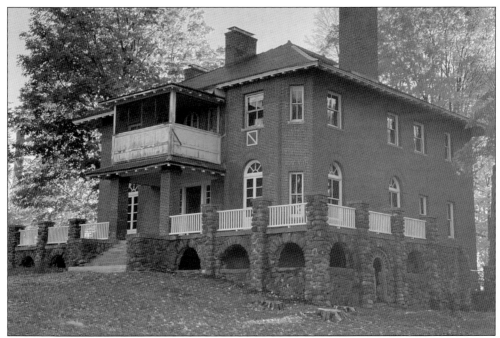

The original Superintendent's Home, known as the Annie G. McDonald Building in honor of the longtime superintendent of nurses, flanks the Old Administration Building on the west. With elements of both Craftsman and Colonial Revival architectural styles, the building boasts an open, balustraded porch with arched fieldstone foundations wrapping around the east and west sides. Inside, the home still possesses its original wooden built-in bookshelves and beautiful brick fireplaces. Vacant for a number of years, the McDonald Building has received recent fame for use in several television shows and motion pictures. (Both, Ashlynn Rickord Werner.)

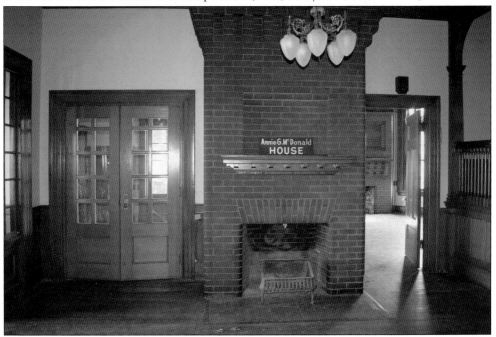

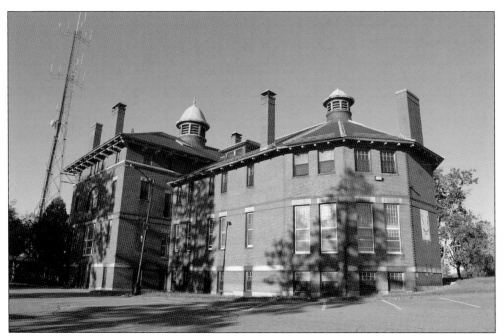

Asylum No. 5, or the Rice Building, sits vacant in the southwest corner of the campus. In the Romanesque Revival style, the building's south side ends in a bay, while the north side features a large, majestic staircase. Patient rooms are unchanged, just empty of furniture and the patients themselves, yet scratch marks are still visible on the insides of the doors. After its closure as an insane hospital for women, the Rice Building later became the Northeast Regional Police Institute, a police in-service training academy, established on March 25, 1983. (Above, Ashlynn Rickord Werner; below, courtesy of David Manch.)

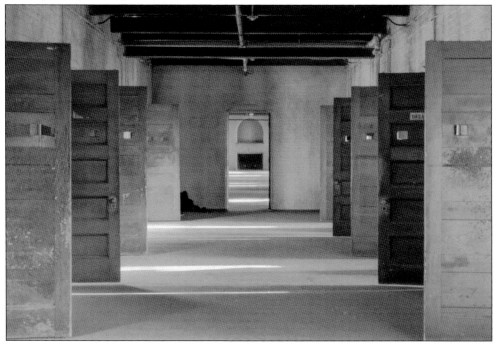

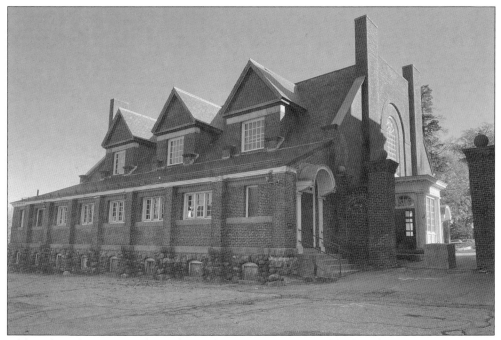

Although no longer actively used for religious services, the Old Chapel continues to serve as a gathering space for Tewksbury Hospital staff and patients, as well as participants in other residential and clinical programs. The kneelers are gone, but an early pulpit and multi-drawered cabinet with a niche for the Communion chalice are indicative of the building's original use. The movie projectors installed in the mid-20th century fill the room on the mezzanine, and the old two-lane bowling alley, long out of use, decays in the basement. (Both, Ashlynn Rickord Werner.)

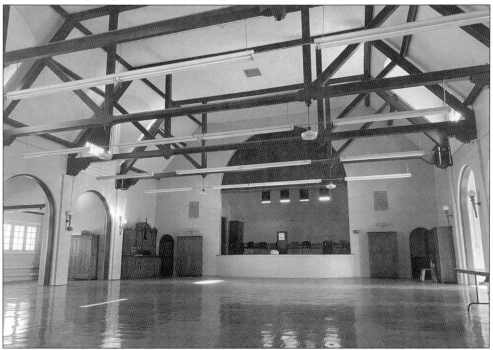

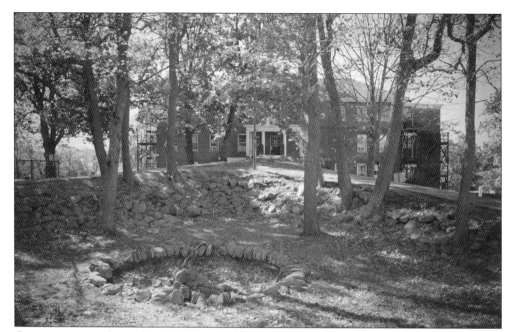

Once serving as a home for nurses, this building remains at the southeast corner of the original quadrangle and looks almost identical to how it did at the turn of the 20th century. The trees have matured, and the fountain is no longer operational, but the structure lives on as the home of MassHealth, an enrollment center in the North Shore. (Ashlynn Rickord Werner.)

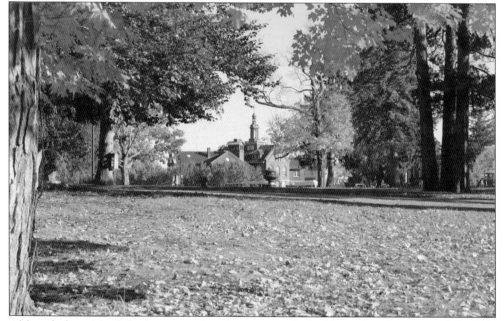

Although the original almshouse quadrangle is missing the buildings that characterized the early institution, the lawn is a remaining element of the historic landscape. Spotted with mature trees likely planted in the late 1800s and early 1900s, the lawn continues to be an inviting space for patients and visitors alike. Note the Anne Sullivan Center, formerly the Hecht Asylum, in the distance. (Ashlynn Rickord Werner.)

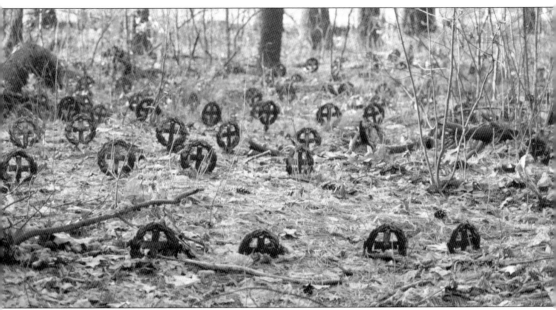

The institution's burial ground came to be known as the Pines Cemetery due to its location amid a pine bank. From the early years as an almshouse, the cemetery was the final resting place for over 10,000 patients at Tewksbury who died between 1854 and the 1930s. Each grave is distinguished with a metal marker, a cross encircled with laurel leaves bearing a number and letter as identification. Although picturesque, the cemetery's location amid hundreds of pine trees and its sheer size has led to extensive debris and overgrowth that have made it hard for visitors to traverse. Local resident Tom Marshall encountered the cemetery for the first time in 2016 while walking his dog along the trail through the woods that contain the Pines Cemetery and set out on a mission to restore it through a community cleanup effort. (Ashlynn Rickord Werner.)

Marshall connected with Joanne Trudelle, longtime Tewksbury Hospital employee and advocate for the cemetery restoration, and they hosted the first cleanup in November 2016. Numerous subsequent cleanups have taken place at the site, along with work to remove dead and dying trees and eradicate poison ivy with funding from the Tewksbury Community Preservation Committee. (Courtesy of Tom Marshall.)

SAVE THE TEWKSBURY HOSPITAL PINES CEMETERY

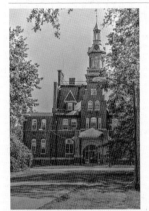

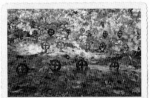

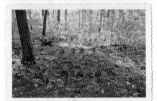

Please join us in cleaning up the Tewksbury Hospital Pines Cemetery at the corner of Livingston and East Streets!

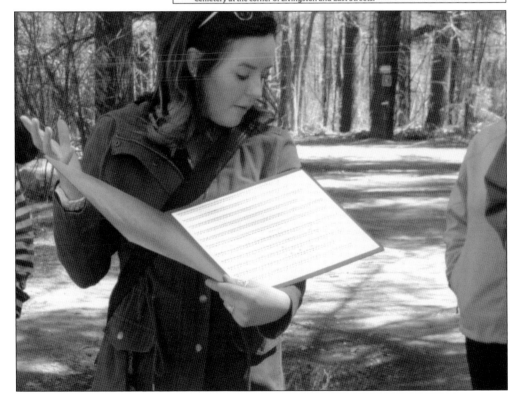

The restoration efforts for the Pines Cemetery are ongoing, with the hope of bringing honor to the thousands who will forever call the cemetery home and their descendants and loved ones who visit the site to pay their respects. The Public Health Museum holds most of the cemetery records and regularly assists visitors in locating the graves of their ancestors. (Ashlynn Rickord Werner.)

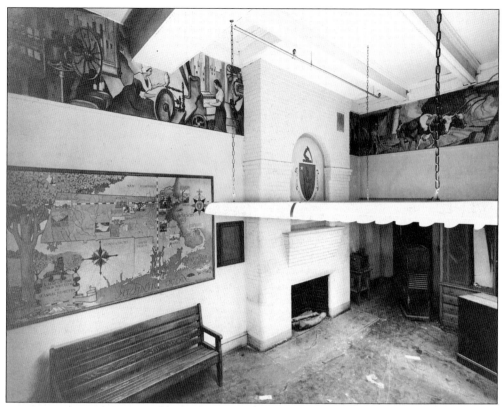

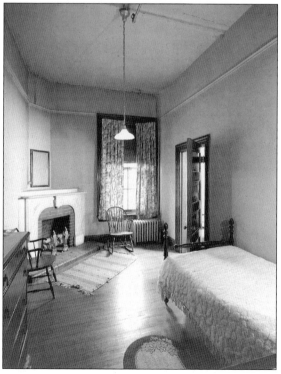

The Public Health Museum in the Old Administration Building interprets the history of the Tewksbury State Hospital as well as other achievements in the field of public health in Massachusetts. Opened on September 30, 1994, the 100th anniversary of the Old Administration Building, the museum's mission is to preserve the past, inspire future practitioners, educate the public, and advance the future of public health through partnerships with various institutions. Occupying multiple rooms on the first floor of the Old Administration Building, the museum boasts a series of murals in the former admitting room, now called the Mural Room, that were completed by members of the Rockport Art Colony in 1934. The museum also exhibited what a typical nurse's room would look like for those who lived on-site.

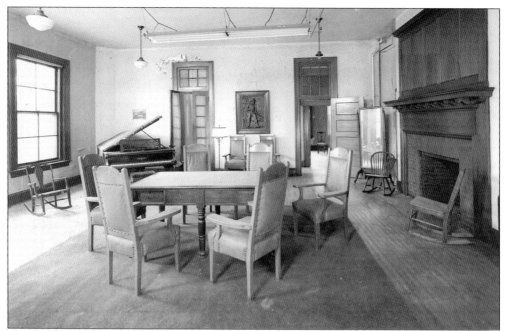

In the early years, the Public Health Museum expected to expand throughout the whole first floor of the Old Administration Building, which included the main offices for the institution's administration as well as the office of the superintendent and the trustees' room. Many of the artifacts on display came from the Tewksbury State Hospital or other area mental hospitals and public health institutions that closed during the latter half of the 20th century. The museum refurbished parts of the building with the help of community members and public health professionals who donated funds to the cause.

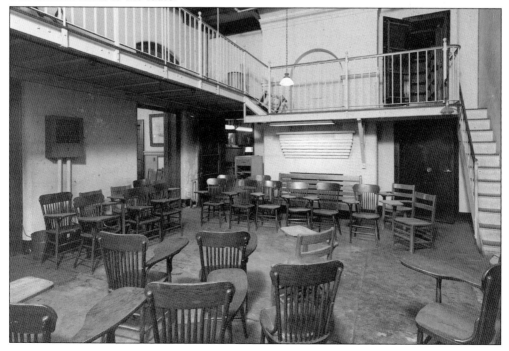

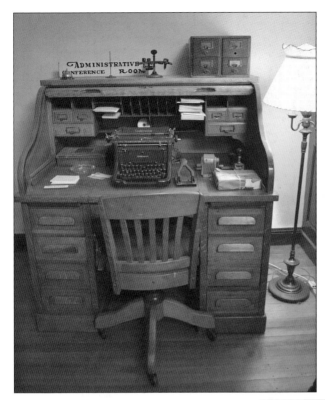

Today, the Public Health Museum presents a range of exhibits covering various public health topics, including the history of the Tewksbury State Hospital. Upon entering the museum, visitors are transported back in time to what a main office of the Old Administration Building would have looked like at the beginning of the 20th century. (Ashlynn Rickord Werner.)

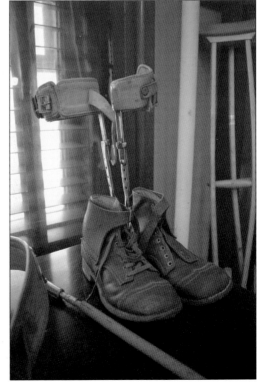

The infectious disease room highlights the history of smallpox, tuberculosis, and polio. A wheelchair, crutches, and these short leg braces act as grim reminders of the epidemic that disproportionately affected children during the mid-20th century before a polio vaccine was introduced and led to the eventual elimination of the disease in the United States. (Ashlynn Rickord Werner.)

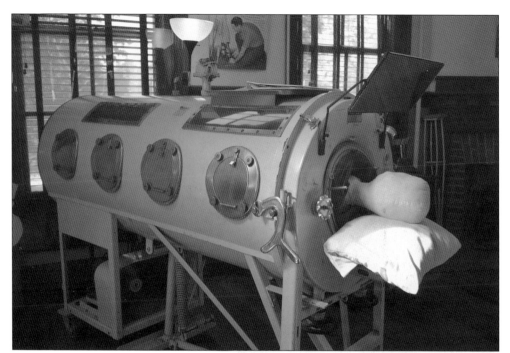

The iron long also accompanies the polio exhibit, a device that provided temporary, but sometimes permanent, breathing support for those with paralysis affecting their ability to breathe. Other exhibits in the infectious disease room include over 100 patent medicine bottles and a display on water sanitation and purification. (Ashlynn Rickord Werner.)

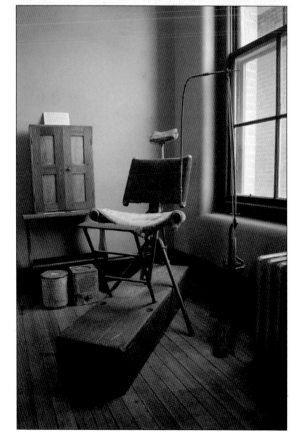

The Public Health Museum also offers exhibits on mental health care and public health nursing, with a focus on the Tewksbury State Hospital. In addition to a series of rotating exhibits in the Mural Room, the museum rounds out with an exhibit on dental health, showcasing a traveling dentist chair and a foot-pedal drill. (Ashlynn Rickord Werner.)

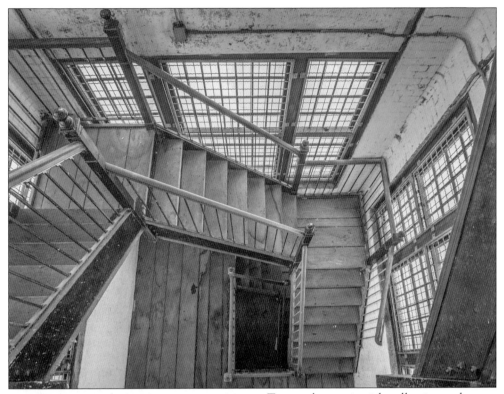

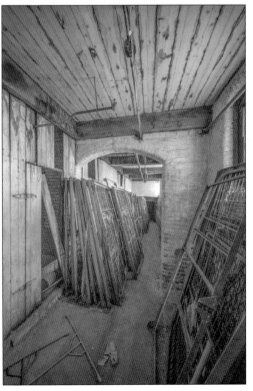

To complement its rich collection and unique location, the Public Health Museum offers regular programming for the community to engage with the history of public health. In addition to lectures and educational events, the museum has hosted photography workshops led by a collaboration between Silver Crescent Photography and Buried By Time Photography since spring of 2019 to document the architecture and history of select buildings at the Tewksbury Hospital. Sites have included the Old Administration Building, the Superintendent's Home, the Rice Building, the Old Chapel, and the greenhouse. As of fall 2020, the partnership has resulted in five successful workshops and over $5,000 donated to the Public Health Museum. (Above, courtesy of David Manch; left, courtesy of Buried By Time Photography Asylum Collection.)

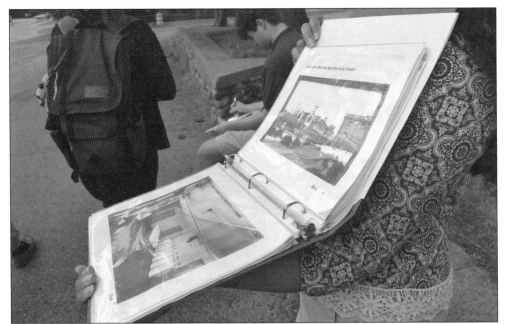

Most notably, the Public Health Museum leads guided walking tours of the Tewksbury State Hospital campus. Visitors explore life in days past, learn about the history of a vibrant community, its architecture, the lives of its patients and staff, and its connection to public health. Most of the images included in this book are shared with tour attendees as they traverse the historic grounds. Stories from Duncan Hazel, an employee of Tewksbury Hospital for 40 years and a longtime museum volunteer before his passing in 2015, are often retold in his memory. When Duncan led a tour, he would share that "there isn't a building here that I haven't been in, under, or through." His passion for documenting the history of the Tewksbury State Hospital provided insight for the writing of this book. (Both, Ashlynn Rickord Werner.)

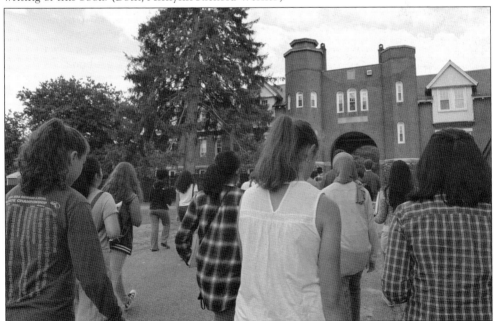

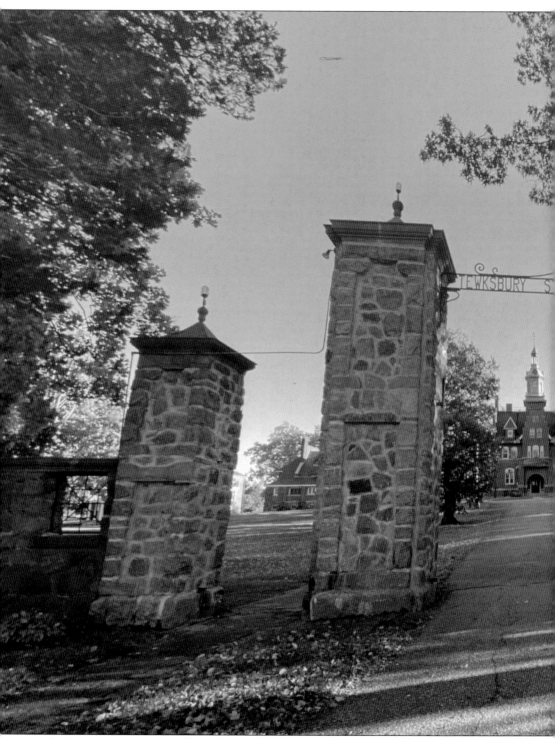

At the center of the town of Tewksbury sits an institution brimming with 700 acres of architectural beauty and a rich history of caring for those in need. While traveling down East Street, it is nearly impossible to miss the impressive stone entrance, looking the same as it did when it was

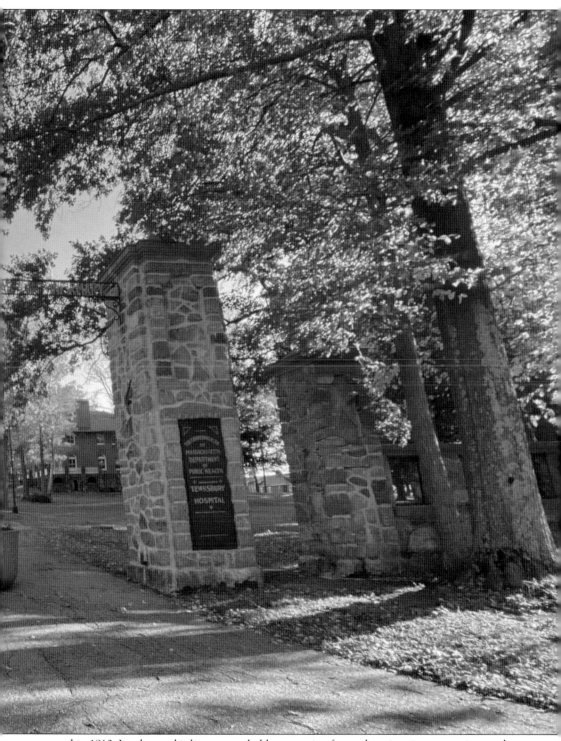

constructed in 1913. Just beyond it lies a remarkable space ripe for exploration, interpretation, and memorialization of all those who have entered through its stone walls. (Ashlynn Rickord Werner.)

Discover Thousands of Local History Books Featuring Millions of Vintage Images

Arcadia Publishing, the leading local history publisher in the United States, is committed to making history accessible and meaningful through publishing books that celebrate and preserve the heritage of America's people and places.

Find more books like this at
www.arcadiapublishing.com

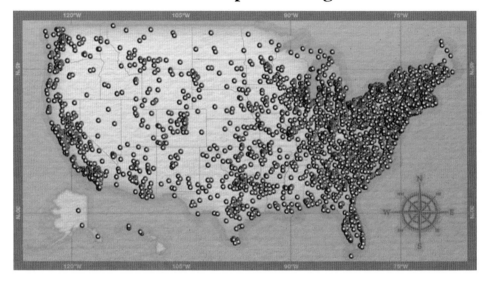

Search for your hometown history, your old stomping grounds, and even your favorite sports team.

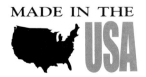